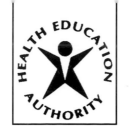

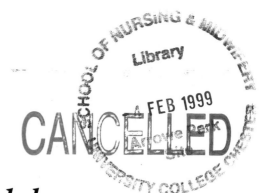

Immunisation: health professionals' information needs – a review of the literature

Volume 2

Helen Bedford, Research Fellow
Department of Epidemiology and Biostatistics
Institute of Child Health
London

Sally Kendall, Professor
Centre for Research in Primary Care Nursing
Buckinghamshire Chilterns University College
Chalfont St Giles
Buckinghamshire

ACKNOWLEDGEMENTS

This immunisation review owes much to the many people whose hard work and help have made it possible. We are very grateful to Dr David Salisbury and Nick Adkin at the Department of Health for their advice, guidance and input; to Plain English Campaign for their contribution; to the reviewers; and to the Health Education Authority's Immunisation Team who have given their full support.

Health Education Authority
Trevelyan House
30 Great Peter Street
London
SW1P 2HW

Printed in England
ISBN 0 7521 0645 7

Contents

Foreword

Ten years ago, immunisation coverage in this country was amongst the lowest third of European countries. Measles epidemics were common with as many as 100,000 reported cases and up to 20 deaths in any one year. Now, coverage is amongst the highest in Europe. New vaccines have been introduced, for example Hib vaccine, with the virtual disappearance of the invasive infections caused by that organism. Epidemics are anticipated and prevented. As we go into the twenty-first century, we can look forward to the global eradication of poliomyelitis, the successful achievement of which will mean that we no longer need to immunise our children against that disease. Measles eradication might follow and with the rapid advances in molecular biology, we can expect new and improved vaccines against infectious and non-infectious diseases.

Whilst there have been considerable operational and technical improvements in immunisation over the last decade, we depend on committed and informed health professionals providing an outstanding service to parents and children. For that service to be most effective, health professionals need to be able to counsel parents in a way that is informative without being patronising, clear and concise, yet taking account of the complex issues that are involved. They must be eloquent in conveying the outstanding personal benefit that children gain through being immunised and the infinitesimally small risks that are attached. In order to undertake this task, health professionals need to understand the tensions that parents face in coming to their decisions. These three volumes provide a detailed account that helps in understanding the factors that contribute to that decision-making process, ranging from the sources of information that are available to parents, to a full enquiry into the circumstances that have contributed to the decisions of a small, but vocal, part of the community to decline immunisation for their children. Within these volumes, the reader will achieve further insight into the interplay between health professional and parent. There will be many important messages.

Those health professionals working in immunisation have much for which they can be rightly proud. With their contribution, we have one of the leading immunisation programmes in the world. Nonetheless, we cannot afford to be complacent and must continually question if the service that we provide is the best possible. The material in these volumes will assist in that task.

DR D M SALISBURY MB BS FRCPCH MFPHM
Head, Immunisation and Infectious Diseases Group
Department of Health, London

2. Background

IMMUNISATION COVERAGE AND INCIDENCE OF INFECTIOUS DISEASE

Immunisation uptake rates in England and Wales are at an all-time high: in March 1996 the average uptake among 2-year-olds of diphtheria, tetanus and polio vaccines was 96%, of pertussis (whooping cough) 94% and of *Haemophilus influenzae* type b (Hib) 95%, while 91% of 2-year-olds had received measles, mumps and rubella (MMR) vaccine.[1] Areas remain, however, where coverage is lower and the range in uptake between districts is 84–100% for third diphtheria, 84–100% for third pertussis and 75–96% for MMR. It is likely that within districts there are even greater variations in uptake between treatment centres.[2]

These high rates have been accompanied by an overall reduction in the incidence of infectious disease, demonstrating the effectiveness of a successful immunisation programme.

- There has been a dramatic decline in notifications of measles, particularly since the introduction of MMR vaccine in 1988.

- A major reduction in the incidence of pertussis has been recorded, with notifications falling from 65,810 to 3963 respectively during the epidemic years of 1982 and 1994, as vaccine coverage has risen.[3]

- Mumps is now considered to be a rare disease in this country.[4]

- The introduction of rubella vaccine has led to an overall decline in the number of rubella infections reported among both children and pregnant women of rubella-associated terminations of pregnancy, and of infants born with congenital rubella syndrome.[5]

From a public health perspective it is important that high coverage rates are maintained to prevent outbreaks of disease. There are many examples of a decline in vaccine coverage resulting in resurgence of disease. These include whooping cough in the late 1970s and early 1980s in England and Wales,[6] diphtheria in the former USSR,[7] and polio among unvaccinated communities in the Netherlands.[8]

FACTORS DETERMINING UPTAKE OF IMMUNISATION

The factors which determine whether a child will be immunised are well established and have been reviewed.[9] These fall into three interrelated categories:

- the enthusiasm and knowledge of health professionals and, in particular, their knowledge of contraindications to immunisation;

- the organisation of the immunisation service itself, including factors at the practice level such as accessibility and, at district level, use of computer databases for evaluating uptake and generating invitations for immunisation;

- parental factors, including social and family issues and attitudes to severity of disease and safety of vaccines.

These determinants of immunisation uptake have been identified largely through quantitative studies. Research using qualitative methods has enabled more detailed exploration of these factors. It provides insights into parents' attitudes, beliefs and experiences of immunisation, and the constraints placed particularly on mothers and how these affect acceptance of immunisation.

References

1. Communicable Disease Surveillance Centre. 'COVER/Körner: January to March 1996', *Communicable Disease Report*, 1996; 6(30): 262.

2. Janes, H. 'Internal variation in the uptake of whooping cough immunisation within a health authority', *Public Health*, 1992; 106: 367–74.

3. White, J.M., Fairley, C.K., Owen, D., Matthews, R.C., Miller, E. 'The effect of an accelerated immunisation schedule on pertussis in England and Wales', *Communicable Disease Review*, 1996; 6(6): R86–R91.

4. Jones, A.G.H., White, J.M., Begg, N.T. 'The impact of MMR vaccine on mumps infection in England and Wales', *Communicable Disease Report*, 1991; 9: R94–R96.

5. Miller, E., Waight, P.A., Vurdien, J.E., Jones, G., Tookey, P.A., Peckham, C.S. 'Rubella surveillance to December 1992: second joint report from the PHLS and National Congenital Rubella Surveillance Programme', *Communicable Disease Report*, 1993; 3: R35–R40.

6. Communicable Disease Surveillance Centre. 'Improvements in the control of whooping cough', *Communicable Disease Report*, 1995; 5(30).

7. Center for Disease Control. 'Diphtheria epidemic - New Independent States of the former Soviet Union, 1990-1994', *Morbidity and Mortality Weekly Report*, 1995; 44(10): 177–81.

8. Oostvoegel, P.M., van Wijngaarden, J.K., van der Avoort, H.G.A.M., Mulders, M.N., Conyn-van Spaendonck, M.A.E., Rumke, H.C. 'Poliomyelitis outbreak in an unvaccinated community in the Netherlands, 1992-93', *The Lancet*, 1994; 344: 665–70.

9. Egan, S., Logan, S. and Bedford, H. *Factors associated with low uptake of immunisation: the role of health education initiatives*. 1992. Unpublished report for the Health Education Authority.

3. The process of immunisation

IMMUNISATION IN THE UK

In the UK the Department of Health (DoH), Welsh Office, Scottish Home and Health Department and DHSS (in Northern Ireland) recommend the following primary immunisations in childhood – a course of three doses of diphtheria, tetanus, pertussis, poliomyelitis and Hib in the first year of life and one dose of MMR vaccine in the second year. As there are neither legal powers to compel uptake nor immunisation requirements for entry to school or other communal groups, parents are free to accept or reject immunisation for their children.

There have been considerable developments in the immunisation programme in recent years. In 1988 combined measles, mumps and rubella (that is, MMR) vaccine was introduced to replace single antigen measles vaccine. MMR vaccine is recommended in the second year of life between 12 and 18 months and, since October 1996, also at 4–5 years. In 1990 the routine schedule for childhood immunisation changed to an accelerated schedule, with immunisation starting at 2 months of age, that is, one month earlier than with the previous schedule. There are now shorter intervals of one month between each of the three doses in the primary course and children complete their course at 4 months of age. In addition, the contraindications to pertussis vaccine have been clarified and, as a consequence of increasing evidence of the safety and benefits of immunisation, there is now a more positive attitude to immunising children who were previously considered to have 'problem histories'. The most recent development was the introduction of Hib vaccine in 1992; this offers infants protection against *Haemophilus influenzae* type b infection, which was the commonest cause of bacterial meningitis in children under 4 years of age in the UK.[1]

If immunisation coverage rates and levels of infectious disease can be taken as measures of the success of these developments, they have been extremely successful. Hib vaccine was introduced in October 1992 and, in 1995, there were 90% fewer laboratory reports of Hib infection (meningitis and septicaemia) in children under 1 year compared with 1992.[2]

It is likely that over the next decade there will be still further developments and improvements in the immunisation programme.[3] These include new vaccines, single-dose combination vaccines, changes to scheduling and the number of doses of vaccine given. For some parents this means that advice and schedules will have changed since their older children were babies and, with more changes in prospect, it is important that parents do not lose confidence in the immunisation programme. To avoid this possibility health professionals need to be equipped with up-to-date information about policy changes and advances.

An example of the implications of developments in the immunisation programme on parents' attitudes emerged in a study by Gill and Sutton (1998) who interviewed 759 mothers with a child aged between 8 and 25 months.[4] The study was conducted in two health districts – a deprived inner-city district with low uptake of immunisation and a more affluent suburban/rural district with a relatively high uptake. It was found that 307 children had completed immunisation courses, while 452 were incomplete; 16% (122) of the mothers said there were immunisations that they would not allow in the future. Of these, 23% said they would not want Hib vaccine and 53% of these said this was because they considered it was untried and untested. The study was conducted at the time of the introduction of Hib vaccine and it is of concern that some parents consider that a new vaccine is untried and untested.

In contrast, the HEA conducts regular waves of research among mothers of children under 3 years old in England. In the past four waves, only 6% have said that there are some immunisations they would not have.[5] Rogers and Pilgrim (unpublished) also found that changes to the programme causes concern for parents, with some mothers considering that the immunisation course now begins too young; one mother had asked the general practitioner (GP) to delay the first immunisation until her child was 6 months old.[6]

INTRODUCING IMMUNISATION

The birth of a baby is notified to the child health services in the relevant health district and this information is forwarded to the health visitor. In most districts the health visitor makes contact with the family when the baby is about 10 days old; prior to this the mother and child are under the care of the midwifery service.[7] The ten-day (or birth) visit may be the first occasion when the subject of immunisation is introduced to parents.

There is little information about the optimum time to introduce the subject of immunisation. In a study of attitudes and knowledge of whooping cough and whooping cough vaccination among 500 parents of young children and expectant parents conducted for the Health Education Council, it was reported that, in general, most parents did not think about immunisation before their child's birth.[8] Following the birth, most parents did not think about whooping cough immunisation (and this can probably be extended to immunisation generally) until the subject was raised by a health professional.

It has been suggested that the antenatal period would be an appropriate time to introduce the subject of immunisation. In a review of parent education, it was pointed out that health professionals have repeatedly observed that women find it hard to think about the period after the birth – labour is seen as a 'brick wall'.[9] In contrast, parents consider that antenatal classes do not provide adequate teaching about childcare. However, it is likely that their views on the appropriate content of antenatal education change after they have given birth. In addition, and of more relevance in this context, local studies show that only a small minority of women (15–28%) attend a full programme of antenatal classes and that they tend to have more advantaged backgrounds.[9] Similarly, although home visits in the antenatal period offer considerable potential for health education, the extent of home visiting during this period by either midwives or health visitors is variable.

Introducing the subject of immunisation at the birth visit may have disadvantages. In the early days and weeks of a child's life, parents have many pressing concerns and are adjusting to the enormous changes which result from a becoming a parent. Immunisation is a major topic and parents may have had little or no time to consider the issue or to prepare questions prior to the health visitor's visit, or may even be unaware that the visit will taking place (an issue that will be explored further later in this review). Recent changes towards a more consumer-led health visiting service mean that in many districts some parents may have very little contact with their health visitor; the birth visit may be one of the few occasions when they are visited at home. This visit provides an important opportunity for introducing the subject and for giving parents written information which they can consult in their own time and discuss later with a health professional.

It is clear that parents want the opportunity for discussion and, as the health visitor is often the first health professional to discuss immunisation with parents, she/he is in a key position of influence. In a detailed study of 82 parents in the North East Thames region, over half the parents interviewed requested an in-depth discussion about immunisation, to be held in private before the immunisations were given.[10] Although parents are invited and encouraged by health visitors to attend child health clinics for advice, weighing and developmental assessment, clinics do not always provide a conducive atmosphere for such detailed discussions. For example, in a study of parents' perceptions of the child health clinic,[11] lack of privacy is suggested as a major area for criticism.

In practice it is likely that the giving of information about immunisation by health professionals is not confined to one consultation. Parents also use a variety of sources of information and, as will be explored later, it is important to ensure that as far as possible they are provided with consistent advice.

CONSENT TO IMMUNISATION

The guidance from the DoH on obtaining consent for immunisation states that consent must always be obtained before immunisation.[12] Consent obtained before the occasion when the child is brought for immunisation is only agreement for the child to be included in the programme. It is not clear to what extent parents or even health professionals understand this distinction. There is no guidance on the information parents should be given before consent to immunisation is sought.

Pearson *et al.* (1993) consider that obtaining consent from parents is a key component of immunisation uptake.[13] Districts differ in their requirements for written consent. In Liverpool, consent to immunisation is sought by the health visitor when the child is 10 days old,[13] whereas in Bath and in Oxford consent for invitation for immunisation for all children born in the district is assumed automatically; negative consent is only entered on to the computer after the invitation is refused and follow-up establishes that the parents do not want their child immunised (*personal communication* – S. Lenton and J. Moreton). In interviews with over 500 mothers conducted for the HEA in 1996,[14] 57% claimed to have been directly asked for their consent to have their child immunised. Of those who had been asked, 90% felt that being asked was important. Interestingly, only 10% of those who were not directly asked for consent considered that it mattered a lot.

Little attention has been paid to the issue of consent to immunisation, for example, what parents and health professionals understand it to be and how and when it is given. In her study of consent to children's heart surgery, Alderson (1990) describes the giving of consent as an ongoing process.[15] This is of particular relevance for immunisation as written consent may be given some weeks before the actual event. Following the change to an accelerated immunisation schedule parents are now required to make a decision about immunisation before their baby is 8 weeks old which, as previously suggested, is in a period when there are many other pressures and concerns. In such circumstances it might be that some parents conform at first to the expectations of the health professionals, wanting to appear to be a 'good parent', and only later have time to consider their actions. Although parents may give their written consent to be included in the programme if requested to do so at the new birth visit, when they receive the invitation to attend for immunisation they have to give consent again by presenting their child at the appointed time. In the intervening period they will have had time to discuss the subject with friends, family and health professionals and will have assimilated information from other sources and will have made a decision taking into account their own experiences with other children.

Information required for consent to immunisation

The UK Government Patient's Charter states that every patient of the National Health Service is 'to be given a clear explanation of any treatment proposed including any risks and alternatives, before deciding whether to agree to the treatment'.[16]

There are no guidelines about precisely what information parents are entitled to be given before deciding whether to have their child immunised. Under English law, patients are only entitled to be told in broad terms the nature and effect of any proposed medical treatment which, in practice, means a doctor need only tell their patient as much or as little as a reasonably competent doctor would be expected to their tell patients. In this situation, those parents who require detailed information of the benefits and risks of immunisation would need to be very well informed and persistent in their questioning.

Deciding what is appropriate information to give parents is complex. In the USA, laws passed in 1992 required the development of vaccine information pamphlets (VIPs) for distribution by health care providers to each parent or carer accompanying a child for immunisation. The purpose is to ensure that parents are provided with sufficient written material concerning the risks and benefits in order to make an informed choice about immunisation. Health care providers who administer the vaccines have to provide copies of the leaflets, and the parent or guardian is required to sign the consent sheet.[17] Since each pamphlet is eight pages long, parents can receive as many as 24 pages of information about immunisation in a single visit. It has been suggested that many parents and physicians thought the leaflets were too detailed and lengthy and dwelt on the risks. A survey of State Health Officials revealed that the information was proving to be a major obstacle to the programme, not only because the information deterred some parents but because of the length of time taken to read the leaflets, particularly if multiple immunisations were taking place.[18]

Clayton *et al.*'s (1994) findings have important implications for the development of information about immunisation in this country.[19] In their study, 375 parents in Nashville were interviewed to determine attitudes and knowledge about immunisation before and after introduction of the VIPs; 198 parents were interviewed before, and 177 after, the pamphlets were introduced. The authors consider the samples had widely differing social and educational backgrounds, although they did not collect information to investigate this claim. The findings showed that parents who received the leaflets knew more about the benefits and minor side-effects of immunisation, and they were also more adamant about accepting immunisation. An interesting additional finding was that the availability of the information did not undermine the parents' perception of health professionals as a source of information. Indeed, receipt of the leaflets made it less likely that parents recalled receiving advice from a source other than health professionals. Although 20% of the parents who received the information said it was too much, others asked for similar information about newer vaccines, such as Hib, for which there was no approved pamphlet. Many parents said it was hard to read all the information at one visit, and expressly asked for it to be provided at an earlier childcare visit so that they had the opportunity to absorb the information in an unhurried setting. In a study of 223 parents surveyed to assess information needs and satisfaction with the VIPs, Fitzgerald and Glotzer (1995) also reported high levels of parental satisfaction among those who were familiar with the leaflets.[20]

Blanket recommendations such as these may not be the most appropriate way forward, however. Fitzgerald and Glotzer's findings[20] support the notion that parents have varied information requirements and that it may not be possible to develop a single information source that addresses the needs of every parent. But, as Mcguire (1990) points out,[21] parents consider that it is the responsibility of the health professionals who are working with them to ensure they receive accurate information which will enable them to make an informed choice about immunisation for their child. Research findings about parents' stated information requirements will be considered in more detail later in this review (see page 28).

PARENTS' VIEWS ABOUT INFORMATION FROM HEALTH PROFESSIONALS

In one of the HEA's regular research waves among mothers of young children in 1996, 70% of mothers said they had discussed immunisation with a health professional before their child's immunisation was due.[14] They were most likely to have consulted a health visitor (52%) or GP (24%). There is, however, considerable evidence that a significant number of parents either think that the amount of information given to them by health professionals is inadequate or do not recall receiving advice at all.[4,6,10,22-5] The HEA commissioned research prior to the introduction of Hib vaccine to determine how the vaccine might be promoted. They used a combination of small group discussions and interviews. Parents viewed advice from health professionals as crucial and they expected GPs and health visitors to provide information on request. However, some parents felt that health professionals did not always have time to give thorough explanations and they felt uneasy about asking questions. The study indicated that a public education campaign can assist in the dialogue between parents and health professionals by raising parents' awareness and providing a basis for their questions.[26]

In a three-part investigation in 1987 of factors influencing uptake of immunisation in Maidstone Health Authority, 174 parents of 13-month-old children were interviewed (with a response rate of 87%).[23] Of these parents, 65% (113) said they lacked knowledge about measles vaccine and 25% expressed uncertainties about possible side-effects. Although measles vaccine was scheduled at 14 months in this district, by the time the children had reached 13 months of age, mothers had received little advice about measles vaccine from health professionals: 92% (160) reported receiving no advice from the child health clinic, 88% (153) no advice from their GP, and 83% (144) no advice from the health visitor. In addition, those who had received advice often found it to be inconsistent. It is acknowledged that, since this study was conducted in 1984, a considerable amount of time and attention has been devoted to the whole issue of immunisation, with training and new guidelines issued regularly. Indeed in their detailed study of 35 mothers, each with a child of 21 months, 48 health visitors and 11 clinical medical officers (CMOs), Mayall and Foster (1989) comment that: 'We had a strong impression that the health worker's position on immunisation had been more carefully worked out and agreed than for other child care topics: health workers had knowledge which they sought to keep updated and they gave parents information on the subject.'[27]

Subsequent studies have also found that parents consider there to be a lack of information from health professionals. In Gill and Sutton's 1993 study of over 700 mothers, 8% said they were dissatisfied with the health professional on their last immunisation visit.[4] Of these, 59% felt they were not told anything at all about immunisation or that they were given inadequate explanations by the health professionals. Two of these parents made comments which express extreme dissatisfaction: 'She offered no information at all. Just did it. She just shoved the needle in' and 'I had to ask about everything. The nurse wasn't very forthcoming about the side-effects, especially as it (Hib) was a new one and I hadn't heard much about it.' While it is acknowledged that these are the comments of only two individuals and cannot therefore be considered representative, it is a cause for concern that any parent has the justification to make such remarks.

Studies that have explored parents' knowledge about immunisation and the reasons why they have not had children immunised also indicate a lack of information. For example, Bennett and Smith (1992)[28] found that parents were not always aware of the timing of immunisations and in Gill and Sutton's study[4] 8% of respondents said they did not know there should be three doses of triple vaccine. Interpreting these findings is difficult but there are several possible conclusions:

- health professionals do not give parents adequate information;

- parents are given information but they forget it, either because it is inadequately communicated or because there is a 'competence gap' that prevents any sharing of decision making,[29] or

- simply that, as a lasting priority, immunisation does not rate very highly and mothers have a lot of other things to think about.

ATTENDANCE FOR IMMUNISATION

As previously discussed, quantitative studies conducted to investigate the determinants of immunisation uptake have identified factors in three interrelated categories. For example, in the national immunisation study,[24] the reasons parents gave for not having their children immunised against measles and pertussis included 'child unwell on the day' (16%), 'time or place inconvenient' (4%), and 'did not attend, no further appointment received' (6%). These point to deficiencies in the immunisation service in that all these children should have been followed up and offered immunisation at a later date. Qualitative research, using information-gathering techniques such as in-depth interviewing, has enabled further exploration of the barriers to immunisation acceptance and findings suggest that they are more complex than they appear.

For example, it has been observed that it is usually the mother who assumes responsibility for child health care.[30] On the day of an immunisation appointment a mother will make an assessment of the situation, including the state of the child's health. If the child often has trivial illnesses and is now well, it is possible the mother may decide not to have her child immunised on that day in case it makes them unwell again (*personal communication* – J. Henderson). Other factors concern the mother's role. These are referred to as gender role constraints, which broadly means a mother has to weigh up the importance of taking a child for an immunisation on that particular day against the difficulties of travelling to the clinic with older children, coping with them in the waiting area, the nagging worry of being late to collect children from school, and the need to perform other essential domestic tasks.[31]

A study of the relationship between transport availability and use of primary health care services by 78 low-income households also describes the complex arrangements individuals often have to make in order to use primary health care services.[32] These observations may be a partial explanation of the finding from a number of studies that children with older siblings are less likely to complete an immunisation course than children in smaller families.[4,10,13,24,31,33] While it is acknowledged that these particular barriers to immunisation uptake go beyond a requirement for improved information, it is important that health professionals recognise the significance of these factors and consider the organisation of services. It is also important to recognise that these factors have relevance for all social groups and not just in households that would be classed as deprived.[31] As one mother commented: 'With three kids it's difficult to keep appointments. It's easier to go on spec, but you can't. The places you take them tend to be small. Try controlling small children in a waiting room, it's not easy. I think they should come to you.'[31]

The venue for immunisation

Under the 1990 GP contract, the method of paying GPs for primary childhood immunisation changed to a system based on the percentage of children on a practice list, aged 2 to 3 years, who have completed courses of immunisation. A large proportion of immunisation provision is carried out in general practice, although this tends to vary according to the type of district.

11

In the national immunisation study of over 3000 parents in 16 districts – 8 with high immunisation coverage (largely rural/suburban) and 8 with low immunisation coverage (largely inner-city) – 70% of immunisations were given in general practice in high uptake districts and 38% in low uptake districts.[24] This finding was confirmed in another study in which data from RICHS (Regional Interactive Child Health System) were used to compare children living in four districts within North East Thames Regional Health Authority.[34] Districts were categorised as rural and suburban or inner-city, with two districts of each type included; 89.8% of 2167 children resident in rural and suburban areas were registered at GP surgeries for immunisation compared with only 38.4% of 1449 children living in inner cities. Both these studies were conducted prior to the introduction of the GP contract and there is little comparable data for the situation since then.

In Gill and Sutton's (1998) study, carried out in 1993, 759 parents were asked about their child's most recent immunisation; 49% had been given at a GP surgery, 26% at the child health clinic, and 24% at combined premises.[4] Although this study was conducted in two contrasting districts, an inner city and an affluent suburban/rural district, the information about immunisation centre was not analysed according to type of district. In the same study parents were asked where they would like to have their child's immunisation done. The response was interesting: 28% would prefer to have it at the GP surgery and given by the GP, 25% would prefer to have their child immunised at home by a health visitor. The range of answers to this question supports the recommendation to provide a flexible service catering for the needs of individual parents.[24,25,35]

Many districts now encourage opportunistic immunisation, not only in general practice and child health clinics but also in hospital accident and emergency departments, and at school, health checks for children who have incomplete immunisation courses.

SUMMARY

- Immunisation rates in England and Wales are at an all-time high but areas remain where coverage is relatively low. To ensure the continued success of the programme extra efforts may be required to maintain high uptake and to improve uptake in other districts.

- There is little information about the optimum time for giving parents information about immunisation. Owing to changes in the schedule, parents have to make a decision soon after a child's birth. Since health visitors have early contact with all families with newborn children they are an important source of information and are valued highly.

- The request for consent to be included in the immunisation programme at ten days after birth maybe unrealistic; parents need information in advance of making this decision.

- Studies show that the majority of parents consider it important for their children to be immunised and are satisfied with their experience of immunisation. A minority have serious criticisms about the service. Parents' dissatisfaction relates to inadequate communication and interpersonal skills on the part of health professionals.

- Parents require encouragement to ask questions and need information before the dialogue with the health professional so that they can consider the issues, formulate questions, and are prepared for a discussion.

- There is no guidance on the minimum amount of information that parents are entitled to receive before consent to immunisation is sought.

- Developments in the immunisation programme, such as changes in contraindications and recommendations for additional doses of vaccines like MMR, may lead some parents to lose confidence in the immunisation programme. More developments are on the horizon and health professionals need to be aware of parents' concerns on this issue.

- A complex interplay of factors may prevent some children from being fully immunised. This highlights the importance of ensuring immunisation service provision is meeting the needs of parents.

References

1. Booy, R., Moxon, E.R. 'Prevention of *Haemophilus influenzae* type b infection by immunisation', *Current Paediatrics*, 1993; 3: 20–3.

2. Communicable Disease Surveillance Centre. 'COVER/Körner: January to March 1966', *Communicable Disease Report*, 1996; 6(30): 262.

3. Salisbury, D.M. 'The future for childhood immunisation', *Current Paediatrics*, 1993; 3: 197–201.

4. Gill, E., Sutton, S. 'Immunisation uptake: the role of parental attitudes' in Hey, V. (ed.) *Immunisation research: a summary volume*. 1998. HEA, London.

5. British Market Research Bureau. Childhood immunisation wave 11. 1996. Unpublished report for the HEA.

6. Rogers, A., Pilgrim, D. 'Non-compliance with childhood immunisation: personal accounts of parents and health care professionals' Unpublished.

7. Goodwin, S. 'Child health services in England and Wales: an overview', *Pediatrics*, (supplement), 1990; 1033–6.

8. MORI. Attitudes towards whooping cough immunisation. 1985. Unpublished report for the HEA, London.

9. Combes, G., Schonveld, A. *Life will never be the same again*. 1992. HEA, London.

10. Pryce, D. Reasons why parents do not present their children for immunisation. 1993. Unpublished report for North East Thames Regional Health Authority.

11. Sefi, S., Grice, D. 'Parents' views of clinics', *Health Visitor*, 1994; 67(20): 62.

12. Department of Health. *Immunisation against infectious diseases*. 1996. HMSO, London.

13. Pearson, M., Makowiecka, K., Gregg, J., Woollard, J., Rogers, M., West, C. 'Primary immunisation in Liverpool, I: who withholds consent?' *Archives of Disease in Childhood*, 1993; 69: 110–14.

14. British Market Research Bureau. *Childhood immunisation survey*. April 1996. Unpublished report for the Health Education Authority.

15. Alderson, P. *Choosing for children*. 1990. Oxford University Press, Oxford.

16. Department of Health. *The patient's charter*. 1991. HMSO, London.

17. Center for Disease Control. 'Publication of vaccine information pamphlets', *Morbidity and Mortality Weekly*, 1991; 40(42): 726–7.

18. Marwick, C. 'Congress to simplify those complex, anxiety-provoking immunisation booklets', *Journal of the American Medical Association*, 1992; 268(24): 3413.

19. Clayton, E.W., Hickson, G.B., Miller, C.S. 'Parents' responses to vaccine information pamphlets', *Pediatrics*, 1994; 93: 369–72.

20. Fitzgerald, T.M., Glotzer, D.E. 'Vaccine information pamphlets: more information than parents want?', *Paediatrics*, 1995; 95(3) 331–4.

21. Mcguire, C. 'Accounting for public perceptions in a childhood immunisation campaign', *Health Education Journal*, 1990; 40(3): 105–7.

22. Blair, S., Shave, N., McKay, J. 'Measles matters, but do parents know?', *British Medical Journal*, 1985; 290: 623–4.

23. Lakhani, A.D.H., Morris, R.W., Morgan, M., Dale, C., Vaile, M.S.B. 'Measles immunisation: feasibility of a 90% target uptake', *Archives of Disease in Childhood*, 1987; 62: 1209–14.

24. Peckham, C., Bedford, H., Senturia, Y., Ades, A. *National Immunisation Study: factors influencing immunisation uptake in childhood*. 1989. Action Research, Horsham.

25. New, S.J., Senior, M.L. '"I don't believe in needles": qualitative aspects of a study into the uptake of infant immunisation in two English health authorities', *Social Science & Medicine*, 1991; 33(4): 509–18.

26. McGuire, C. 'The *Haemophilus influenzae* type b (Hib) vaccine: a pre-launch qualitative study of parental perceptions', *Health Education Journal*, 1992; 51(4): 171–5.

27. Mayall, B., Foster, M.C. *Child health care: living with children, working for children*. 1989. Heinemann Nursing, Oxford.

28. Bennett, P., Smith, C. 'Parents' attitudes towards immunisation in Wales according to socio-economic group: a preliminary investigation', *Health Education Journal*, 1992; 51(3): 127–31.

29. Watson, E., Sim, J. 'The health visitor's visit', *Health Visitor*, 1989; 62(7): 214–17.

30. Graham, H. *Women, health and the family*. 1984. Health Education Council/Harvester Press, Brighton.

31. Senior, M.L., New, S.J., Gatrell, A.C., Francis, B.J. 'Geographic influences on the uptake of infant immunisations: 2. Disaggregate analyses', *Environment and Planning A*, 1993; 25: 467–79.

32. Pearson, M., Dawson, C., Moore, H., Spencer, S. 'Health on borrowed time? Prioritizing and meeting needs in low-income households', *Health and Social Care*, 1993; 1: 45–54.

33. Li, J., Taylor, B. 'Childhood immunisation and family size', *Health Trends*, 1993; 25(1): 16–19.

34. Li, J., Taylor, B. 'Comparison of immunisation rates in general practice and child health clinics', *British Medical Journal*, 1991; 303: 1035–8.

35. Nicoll, A., Elliman, D., Begg, N.T. 'Immunisation: causes of failure and strategies and tactics for success', *British Medical Journal*, 1989; 299: 808–12.

4. Health professionals

ROLES IN IMMUNISATION PROVISION

Health visitors

Health visitors are broadly concerned with the promotion of health and prevention of ill health and, as their work is mainly focused on families with preschool children, they have a key role in childhood immunisation. They have been shown to be the main advisers to parents about immunisation,[1-3] so it is of concern that some parents do not recall receiving any advice from them. One study reported 44% of respondents saying they had not been given verbal information from their health visitor, and only 57% said they had received written information about immunisation.[4]

Despite this, Mayall and Foster (1989) identified service orientation to immunisation as a model of how child health services in general should be offered.[5] They found that parents and health visitors were largely in agreement over their respective roles and responsibilities: it is the responsibility of health visitors to provide parents with information about immunisation and parents have the final decision whether to accept immunisation. About one-third of the health visitors viewed their role as providing information to parents and giving them the opportunity to discuss the issue (the CMOs also took this view). Most health visitors believed their role was to encourage uptake of immunisation, and this varied from mild encouragement, to pushing, and to chasing up defaulters. It was interesting to note that, even health visitors who the authors described as 'prescriptive' and 'authoritarian' regarding other health topics adopted a softer style when discussing immunisation. This was explained as being partly due to 'the controversial pertussis vaccine'.

Discussing pertussis vaccine in particular can be difficult for some health visitors, and one commented that the more information she was exposed to, especially from television programmes, the more unsure she became about discussing it with parents. Such concerns have been expressed elsewhere. In a study of 106 health visitors' views on immunisation in Oxfordshire,[1] nearly half of the health visitors admitted to worrying about the advice they gave to parents on immunisation. This was not found to be a reflection of whether they felt they needed updating. It is probably partly a consequence of occasional adverse publicity about immunisation. (This will be discussed on page 20.)

Only three health visitors in Mayall and Foster's study[5] explicitly mentioned having a public health role in relation to immunisation and they acknowledged this might create conflicts of interest: while they were concerned for the child population as a whole, parents were concerned for their own, particular, loved child. This is an important consideration in planning the content of information for parents.

Much debate has concerned health visitors increasing their role and being provided with the training and encouragement to give immunisations. This has been put forward as one method of ensuring that children from hard-to-reach families are provided with the immunisation service in the home setting.[2] Arguments in favour of such a development are

- as nurses, health visitors are competent to perform such a task;
- the health promotion message is reinforced if it is accompanied by immunisation;
- health visitors should address the needs of their clients, where necessary providing a home immunisation service.

However, there have also been strong arguments against health visitors taking on this task:

- providing immunisation in the home may encourage misuse of services;
- it would detract from health visitors' role as health promoters;
- there is adequate provision for families already;
- health visitors are fearful of managing severe adverse reactions, such as anaphylaxis, in the home.[6,7]

In a study of health visitors in 20 districts,[8] only 17% of respondents said they would be willing to give immunisations in the home without a doctor present. However, the proportion willing to take on this task appears to vary from district to district since 64% of health visitors surveyed in Oxfordshire were prepared to give immunisation to children in the home without a doctor present.[1] Increasingly, trusts are providing both the training and support for health visitors to give immunisation.

Begg and White's 1988 survey of preschool immunisation programmes in England and Wales involved collecting information from 183 districts about the administrative, nursing and medical aspects of the immunisation programme.[9] In 21% of the districts health visitors were routinely giving immunisations. Evaluation of a domiciliary immunisation service where immunisation is given by a specially trained nurse has shown it to be an acceptable, cost-effective and effective means of providing immunisation,[10] and it appears to have other benefits. Health visitors who provide a domiciliary service in Newcastle reported that immunising a child in the home often gives mothers the confidence to attend the clinic for the rest of the immunisation course, and it increases trust and demonstrates to the parent that the health visitor is really interested in their child.[11]

Practice nurses

In Gill and Sutton's 1993 study parents were asked who had given their child's most recent immunisation.[4] It had been given by a nurse in 40% of cases, by a doctor in 54% of cases (GP 30%, clinic doctor 24%), and by a health visitor in 4% of cases. This finding reflects the increasing tendency for nurses employed within general practice to perform this type of task. The number of practice nurses has increased since the introduction of the GP contract – DoH figures show that in 1988 there were about 7000 practice nurses and about 18,000 by the end of 1991.[12]

Several studies, which have explored the nature of work undertaken by practice nurses either by surveying the nurses themselves[13-15] or by investigating GPs' expectations,[16] confirm that practice nurses have a major involvement in childhood immunisation. Despite this, Gill and Sutton found that only 4% of respondents in their study would seek advice from the practice nurse about immunisation.[4] However, this may be because they were only seen in the context of giving injections, and thus at a stage when a parent had already made the decision to have their child immunised. In some districts clinic nurses and district nurses may also be involved in giving childhood immunisations.[8]

In a study of 899 practice nurses in South West Thames Regional Health Authority, 76% of the 620 respondents reported being currently involved in childhood immunisation.[15] Of these, 14.5% had completed a post-registration course in practice nursing and a further 5.8% were qualified health visitors. Interestingly, the authors also reported that the majority of the practice nurses surveyed wished to develop their role in counselling/communication skills and health promotion. This may partly reflect the effect of the GP contract on the working culture of general practice and the recognition of the importance of counselling skills as health promotion assumes a greater role. Patients too consider communication skills are important, rating them as the most sought-after quality of the primary care provider.[17]

General Practitioners and Clinical Medical Officers

Studies suggest that the doctor's role in immunisation is highly valued by parents. In Gill and Sutton's study the majority of the most recent immunisations had been given by a doctor.[4] In addition, GPs were the health professionals whom parents would be most likely to ask for information about immunisation (51%) and would prefer to give their child's next immunisation (28%). This finding was despite the dearth of information that had actually been given by GPs, since only 37% of respondents had received any verbal advice from their GP and only 17% written information.

Since the introduction of the GP contract, there have been anecdotal reports, as well as evidence from qualitative studies, indicating that some parents are being put under pressure to have their children immunised in order that GPs may meet the targets for payment.[18] There have also been reports of parents being excluded from GPs' lists if they refuse immunisation (*personal communication* – Community Nursing Adviser, Royal College of Nursing). This was confirmed by a detailed study of the views of 58 health professionals on varying aspects of immunisation. One GP felt his relationship with patients was being damaged because of target payments. Some of the health professionals described GPs telling parents that unless their child was vaccinated they should register with another GP, or refusing to register these children.[19] This is a major cause for concern. Unfortunately, because of the target payment system, some parents consider that GPs are unlikely to provide an objective view about immunisation,[4,20] while health visitors may be viewed as being more impartial.

Clinical Medical Officers, usually working from community child health clinics, are important providers of immunisation and of advice about immunisation. As already noted, many parents attend child health clinics for immunisation and for preventive child health services generally and, in their child's early years, may have more contact with the CMO than with their own GP, thus developing a close and trusting relationship.

Primary health care team

In the national immunisation study,[2] a team approach to immunisation where all members of the primary health care team shared responsibility for immunisation provision, was found to have a beneficial effect on immunisation uptake. It is not difficult to appreciate that such an approach, with enthusiastic health professionals working together to provide a flexible service and giving consistent advice, will prove successful. This has been borne out in practice, where adopting such an approach has ensured high uptake rates even in deprived inner city districts.[21,22] Research has not usually considered the role of clerical and nursing support staff in general practice and community clinics. They too have an important role to play and should be included in any training so that they are familiar with the aims of the immunisation service.

Other health professionals

In addition to the health professionals who are providing information and giving immunisations, there are other individuals whose activities are essential for the running of a successful immunisation programme within a district. The programme is generally coordinated by the District Immunisation Coordinator.[23] Others involved include community physicians, paediatricians, consultants in communicable disease control, community unit administrators, health educators and pharmacists. With districts increasingly adopting policies of opportunistic immunisation, in hospitals and schools for example, other health professionals such as hospital nurses, medical house officers and school health nurses have become involved in the provision of immunisation.

HEALTH PROFESSIONALS' ATTITUDES AND KNOWLEDGE ABOUT IMMUNISATION

Knowledge

One of the key factors determining high uptake of immunisation is the health professionals' knowledge about the contraindications to immunisation. In the national immunisation study, GPs' knowledge was found to be directly associated with the level of uptake in their practice.[2] Studies that have either directly assessed health professionals' knowledge[1,2,24-7] or investigated the reasons parents gave for non-immunisation,[28-31] have demonstrated that some health professionals are poorly informed about the contraindications to immunisation. There is no comparable information on the level of knowledge about contraindications to immunisation since the introduction of Hib vaccine and the most recent edition of the DoH memorandum on immunisation.[32]

It is essential that health professionals are well informed about the contra-indications to immunisation, not only because children may be inappropriately denied protection but also because children who have valid contraindications (very few in practice) may be inappropriately immunised. In addition, there have been many reports of parents being given conflicting advice about whether their child should be immunised – a situation which may lead to parental confusion and loss of confidence in health professionals generally. It is also important to remember that the changes in advice which result from alterations in immunisation schedules and recommendations may be perceived by parents as being conflicting.

For example, in their report of three years' experience in a specialist advisory service for immunisation in Leeds, Newport and Conway (1993) state that in 78% (46) of cases referred to the clinic there was agreement between the referring doctor and the clinic about whether the child should be immunised.[33] Despite correct interpretation on the part of the GPs, referral was still thought necessary either because the parent wanted a second opinion or because the GP required confirmation of their decision in a difficult case. The authors consider an important factor in parents' need for a specialist opinion to be previous conflicting advice, and that the GP's correct advice had only added to parental confusion.

Attitudes

Health professionals' attitudes to immunisation, as determined by their perceptions about the severity of disease and safety and efficacy of vaccines, have also been explored. In the national immunisation study of 1793 GPs, health visitors, CMOs and paediatricians,[2] the overwhelming majority of health professionals were positive about immunisation and 97% said they encouraged measles and pertussis immunisation. In this study, health professionals' attitudes in themselves were found to have no particular influence on immunisation uptake but this is probably because the vast majority of health professionals expressed positive attitudes. However, parents' reports suggest that attitudes are not always transmitted; 62% and 56% respectively of respondents to a later study thought their health visitor and their GP considered it was extremely important for young children to have their immunisations. Almost a quarter (23%) did not know what their health visitor's attitude was, and 38% did not know their GP's attitude.[4]

HEALTH PROFESSIONALS' INFORMATION NEEDS

There is a paucity of research with the specific aim of exploring health professionals' information needs with respect to immunisation. Prior to the Hib campaign, the HEA commissioned a qualitative study among health professionals in England to explore their awareness of Hib and their information needs regarding the new vaccine to be launched in 1992.[34] Three districts with different immunisation coverage rates were selected and in-depth interviews were conducted in each district with the immunisation coordinator, community paediatrician and health promotion manager. Additionally, a total of four GP practices/child health clinics in each district were visited and the relevant staff involved in immunisation (GPs/CMOs, practice/clinic nurses, health visitors) were interviewed in depth. A total of 40 interviews were achieved in all.

The study revealed very positive attitudes towards immunisation and commitment towards improving immunisation rates. Health professionals' information requirements with respect to the new vaccine included detailed information on Hib itself, trial data, details of the vaccine, contraindications, side-effects, effect of combining Hib with other vaccines, clear details of the schedule and catch-up programmes, and practical details such as cost and purchase source. Importantly, health professionals wanted the information several months in advance of the introduction of the vaccine so that they could be fully prepared. Training was viewed as crucial to provide a consistent message to parents both nationally and at practice/clinic level.

The health professionals were asked about the most appropriate means of communicating the information. The doctors expected to see features about Hib in their professional journals – the *British Medical Journal* and the *Journal of the Royal College of General Practitioners* – as well as the popular medical press – *Pulse*, *GP* and *Doctor*. Health visitors and nurses would see articles from other magazines as well as reading their own professional journals.[34]

Implications of adverse publicity about immunisation

The speed of development in the immunisation programme, together with occasional adverse publicity about immunisation, for example pertussis vaccine in the 1970s, increases the demands by parents for information. Health professionals need to have readily available and up-to-date information in order to answer the inevitable queries that parents raise.

For example, in a paper published in *The Lancet* it was suggested that measles vaccine was associated with Crohn's disease.[35] This attracted considerable publicity in both the press and on television. Other papers and correspondence which do not support these claims, published both before and subsequently, were not well publicised.[36-9] Since some of these were published in less widely read scientific journals to which there may be limited access, many health professionals may be unaware that this important information is available. In this situation health professionals are little better informed than the parents who are seeking advice; anxieties have been raised but health professionals are poorly equipped through lack of information to allay fears. At times of adverse publicity they need extra support and all the relevant information quickly so that they are equipped to answer parents' questions.

SUMMARY

- Health visitors have been identified as having a major role in providing information and encouraging uptake of immunisation. In many districts they have extended their role to include giving immunisations. This is a very valuable development and is particularly useful for hard-to-reach families.

- Some health visitors find discussing aspects of immunisation difficult, particularly pertussis vaccine, and worry about the advice they give parents.

- Practice nurses are an important group to consider; they have grown in number and have an increasingly important role in giving immunisation. They are keen to enhance their communication/counselling skills.

- The role of GPs is valued by parents and they are the source of advice most parents would consult. However, as a result of the GP contract which provides payment for reaching target levels of uptake, they are perceived by some parents as unlikely to give impartial advice.

- There is a lack of recent research investigating professionals' knowledge about immunisation. Since this is such an important factor in achieving immunisation targets, and in the light of the rapid developments in the immunisation programme, consideration should be given to undertaking regular assessments of health professionals' knowledge.

- There is a dearth of research specifically investigating health professionals' information needs with respect to immunisation.

References

1. Robertson, C.M., Bennett, V.J. 'Health visitor's views on immunisation', *Health Visitor*, 1987; 60: 221–2.

2. Peckham, C., Bedford, H., Senturia, Y., Ades, A. *National Immunisation Study: factors influencing immunisation uptake in childhood*. 1989. Action Research, Horsham.

3. Carter, H., Jones, I.G. 'Measles immunisation: results of a local programme to increase vaccine uptake', *British Medical Journal*, 1985; 290: 1717–19.

4. Gill, E., Sutton, S. 'Immunisation uptake: the role of parental attitudes' in Hey, V. (ed.) *Immunisation research: a summary volume*. 1998. HEA, London.

5. Mayall, B., Foster, M.C. *Child health care: living with children, working for children*. 1989. Heinemann Nursing, Oxford.

6. Thompson, J. 'Immunisation and the health visitor' (letter), *The Lancet*, 1984; i: 517.

7. Rogers, S. 'Health visitors' bottom line', *Nursing Times*, 1988; 84(28): 15.

8. British Market Research Bureau. 'The uptake of pre-school immunisation in England.' 1989. Unpublished report for the Department of Health.

9. Begg, N., White, J. 'A survey of pre-school immunisation programmes in England and Wales.' 1988. *Community Medicine* 10:344–50.

10. Jefferson, N., Sleight, G., Macfarlane, A. 'Immunisation of children by a nurse without a doctor present', *British Medical Journal*, 1987; 294: 423–4.

11. Waterson, T. 'Health visitors' experience of immunisation', *Community Paediatric Group Newsletter*, 1993.

12. Sheppard, J. 'The clinical task', in Pringle, M. (ed.) *Change and teamwork in primary care*. 1993. British Medical Journal, London.

13. Bradford J. M., Winn, S. 'A survey of practice nurses' views of health promotion', *Health Education Journal*, 1993; 52(2): 91–5.

14. Peter, A. 'Practice nursing in Glasgow after the new general practitioner contract', *British Journal of General Practice*, 1993; 43: 97–100.

15. Ross, F.M., Bower, P.J., Sibbald, B.S. 'Practice nurse: characteristics, workload and training needs', *British Journal of General Practice*, 1994; 44: 15–18.

16. Robinson, G., Beaton, S., White, P. 'Attitudes towards practice nurses – survey of a sample of general practitioners in England and Wales', *British Journal of General Practice*, 1993; 43: 25–9.

17. Drury, M., Greenfield, S., Stilwell, B., Hull, F.M. 'A nurse practitioner in general practice: patient perceptions and expectations', *Journal of Royal College of General Practitioners*, 1988; 38: 503–5.

18. Forrest, J. *Who calls the shots? An analysis of lay beliefs about childhood vaccination.* Occasional Paper in Sociology and Social Policy No. 3: 1995. South Bank University, London.

19. Alderson, P., Mayall, B., Barker, S., Henderson, J., Pratten, B. 'Childhood immunisation: meeting targets yet respecting consent.' *European Journal of Public Health,* 1997; 7: 95–100.

20. Rogers, A., Pilgrim, D. 'Non-compliance with childhood immunisation: personal accounts of parents and health care professionals' Unpublished.

21. Ross, S.K. 'Childhood immunoprophylaxis: achievements in a Glasgow practice', *Health Bulletin,* 1983; 41(5): 253–7.

22. Toon, P.D. 'Achieving immunisation targets in an inner city practice', *Maternal and Child Health,* February 1992: 42–4.

23. Crittenden, P., Rao, M. 'The immunisation coordinator: improving uptake of childhood immunisation', *Communicable Disease Report,* 1994; 4: R79–R81.

24. Hull, D. 'Interpretation of the contraindications to whooping cough vaccination', *British Medical Journal,* 1981; 283: 1231–3.

25. Wilkinson, J.R. 'Measles immunisation – contraindications perceived by general practitioners in one health district', *Public Health,* 1986; 100: 144–8.

26. Lakhani, A.D.H., Morris, R.W., Morgan, M., Dale, C., Vaile, M.S.B. 'Measles immunisation: feasibility of a 90% target uptake', *Archives of Disease in Childhood,* 1987; 62: 1209–14.

27. Berkeley, M.I.K. 'The effect of attitudes on immunisation', *Health Bulletin,* 1983; 41(3): 141–4.

28. Adjaye, N. 'Measles immunisation: some factors affecting non-acceptance of vaccine', *Public Health,* 1985; 95: 185–8.

29. Stevens, D., Baker, R. 'Parents' beliefs about vaccination', *British Medical Journal,* 1989; 299: 257.

30. Klein, N., Morgan, K., Wansborough-Jones, M.H. 'Parents' beliefs about vaccination: the continuing propagation of false contraindications', *British Medical Journal,* 1989; 298: 1687.

31. Barlow, H., Walker, D. 'Immunisation in Fife part II – failure to immunise against whooping cough – reasons given by parents, *Health Education Journal,* 1990; 49(3): 103–5.

32. Department of Health. *Immunisation against infectious diseases.* 1996. HMSO, London.

33. Newport, M.J., Conway, S.P. 'Experience of a specialist service for advice on childhood immunisation', *Journal of Infection,* 1993; 26: 295–300.

34. MORI. 'The Hib vaccine – exploring information needs among health professionals'. 1992. Unpublished report for the HEA, London.

35. Thompson, N.P., Montgomery, S.M., Pounder, E.R., Wakefield, A.J. 'Is measles vaccination a risk factor for inflammatory bowel disease?', *The Lancet,* 1995; 345: 1071–4.

36. Gilat, T., Hacohen, D., Lilos, P., Langman, M.J.S. 'Childhood factors in ulcerative colitis and Crohn's disease: an international co-operative study', *Scandinavian Journal of Gastroenterology,* 1987; 22: 1009–24.

37. Iizuka, M., Nakagomi, O., Chiba, M., Ueda, S., Masamune, O. 'Absence of measles virus in Crohn's disease', *The Lancet,* 1995; 345: 199.

38. Farrington, P., Miller, E. 'Measles vaccination as a risk factor for inflammatory bowel disease', *The Lancet,* 1995; 254: 1362.

39. Haga, Y., Funakoshi, O., Kuroe, K., Kanazawa, K., Nakajima, H., Saito, H. *et al.* 'Absence of measles viral genomic sequence in intestinal tissues from Crohn's disease by nested polymerase chain reaction', *Gut,* 1996; 38(2): 211–15.

5. Parents' attitudes, beliefs and perceptions

THE DECISION TO IMMUNISE

It is well established that parents' attitudes are an important determinant of immunisation acceptance, in particular, perceptions of the severity of infectious disease and whether it is viewed as a threat.[1] For example, despite its association with significant morbidity and even death, measles is regarded by some individuals as 'almost a normal incident in an English childhood'.[2] Diseases that are considered to be more serious, such as polio and diphtheria, are now so rare in this country that they are not perceived to be an imminent threat.[3,4] Perceptions about the safety and efficacy of vaccines are also crucially important as the experience of the whooping cough vaccine controversy in the 1970s demonstrated. The overall decline in infectious disease may lead to a greater concern about the possible risks of the vaccines.

The way in which attitudes to immunisation are formed and how the decision whether or not to accept immunisation for a child is made are little understood. Qualitative research[5] and anecdotal evidence indicates that there is a wide interplay of influences on parents. For example, a detailed study of 33 mothers who each had a child aged 21 months described how mothers' knowledge of immunisation came from a variety of sources: relatives, friends, leaflets, magazines and the media.[6] Most mothers reported discussions with health professionals, mainly health visitors, but also CMOs, GPs, hospital doctors, medical friends and homeopaths. This finding is confirmed by other studies that have investigated parents' sources of information.[1,3,7]

Clearly the quality of information provided and the effectiveness with which it is communicated are crucial factors in the decision-making process and, as has been discussed already, there is considerable evidence that information from health professionals is often lacking or inconsistent. New and Senior (1991),[8] however, consider that, regardless of the levels of professional advice received, most mothers base their decision about immunisation, at least in part, on a wide range of past experiences which seem to exert a far stronger influence than the empirical evidence offered to them by health professionals in support of immunisation. Nevertheless, there is considerable room for health professionals to improve their information-giving skills. Communication training could help in this respect and could also enable them to elicit information about past experiences and outside influences and respond to them appropriately, thus making their advice more influential in the decision-making process.

A number of studies demonstrate how cultural background, belief systems and previous personal experience in both childhood and as a parent are important influences on the decision to immunise. In interviews with 135 mothers with children aged between 18 and 36 months, 51% of the children were reported to be fully immunised.[9] Reasons for non-immunisation included fear of pertussis vaccines and medical reasons. There were differences between socio-economic groups in both take-up of vaccines and reasons given for non-acceptance, with lower uptake of pertussis and measles vaccine in socio-economic groups IV and V than in I and II. Interestingly, mothers in the more socio-economically deprived groups were also more likely to cite a medical reason for their refusal (40% in IV and V compared with 14–17% in higher groups), suggesting that lower social groups felt their refusal needed to be justified more strongly and they could not simply refuse. The authors commented that mothers found the decision whether or not to have their child immunised extremely difficult.

Attitudes to pertussis immunisation among 228 parents in Wales were explored by Bennett and Smith (1992) who found that 128 parents had at some time either delayed immunisation or made a decision not to have the immunisation.[10] Worries over a child's distress after having the injection were important or very important factors in the decision of 49% of this group not to have further immunisations; 61% expressed the same level of concern relating to short-term illness. In addition, nearly a fifth of parents who had delayed or decided not to immunise their child reported that previous unsympathetic treatment by clinic staff was a factor in their decision. The authors conclude that a significant percentage of parents who fail to complete or start immunisation programmes are unlikely to be influenced simply by repeated requests to attend, which may be interpreted by parents as harassment. This observation has been confirmed by Rogers and Pilgrim (unpublished).[4] These parents appear to be anxious about the risks, underestimate the benefits of immunisation, and may also be reacting to negative experiences of the immunisation process itself.

The development of the decision to immunise

The view that the decision to have a child immunised is a developing process is further supported by mothers' accounts of how they decided to have their first-born children immunised. For many it was an automatic process, while for subsequent children it was often not so straightforward. An example of this emerged in New and Senior's detailed study[8] of 253 women in north-west England which included 123 full immunisers (child had received the full course of DTP – diphtheria, tetanus and pertussis – and polio), 71 partial immunisers (child had received the full course minus pertussis vaccine), and 48 incomplete immunisers (child had not completed a course, irrespective of whether pertussis vaccine was included). Amongst the incomplete immunisers, one mother had been put off taking her children for immunisation because her eldest son had developed an allergy following his first injection. She had been told that he would not suffer any side-effects, but as she perceived he had done so she was understandably suspicious of the advice given to her by health professionals.

There is conflicting evidence about 'immunisation running in families', that is, if an older child receives pertussis vaccine whether or not it is more likely that their younger siblings will also receive the vaccine. Gill and Sutton (1998) found a strong relationship between a child having completed a course of pertussis vaccine and their older sibling/s having also done so.[3] In contrast, in their study of the relationship of socio-economic variables and consent to immunisation in Liverpool, Pearson *et al.* (1993) found that parents were less likely to give consent for pertussis vaccine for children with older siblings.[11] The authors consider this may reflect a cohort effect associated with parental experience of either older children reacting to pertussis vaccine or little experience of whooping cough disease. However, as this study was not able to investigate whether or not parents had actually consented to pertussis vaccine for their older children, it is not possible to draw any firm conclusions. Another interesting finding from this study, which is difficult to interpret, was that parents were less likely to consent to pertussis vaccine for boys than for girls.

Rogers and Pilgrim's (unpublished) in-depth study provides useful information about the attitudes and experiences of a small group of highly motivated mothers who decided not to have their children immunised.[4] The study sample was small (19) and self-selected; although information is not included in their report on how the sample was selected, it is understood that an advertisement was placed in *The Informed Parent* (issue 2, 1993), the publication of a parents' support group of the same name, asking for interested parents to contact the researchers. It is of particular interest that all but five of these women had started as immunisers and only later became non-compliers, adding further support to the notion of the immunisation decision being a developing process. For these mothers information and experience had given them critical insights which they lacked when they encountered immunisation for the first time as new parents. As in previous studies this partly resulted from children's immunisation reactions. Five of the mothers reported side-effects which they considered went beyond the 'mild' symptoms they had been advised about by health professionals. They were also influenced by reports of side-effects from friends and other mothers they met at informal support groups.

A further study reported that 13% (90) of parents said they had problems with their child's most recent immunisation in terms of side-effects; of these, 21% said they had been distressed by quite severe reactions – including children who were 'irritable, screaming and distressed' (7%), had a 'raging temperature' (4%), were 'admitted to hospital' (3%), or 'had convulsions' (2%).[3]

Individual or public health perspective?

These studies highlight the concern many parents have about reactions to immunisation. While the message promoted by the DoH and HEA is that children should be immunised to protect them against infectious disease, it is evident that some parents think in terms of protecting their child from the pain of the injection and distress of a reaction, particularly if they have a dislike of injections themselves. This is a further example of the differing perspectives of immunisation, public health versus individual.

It is important for health professionals to recognise that the severity of a reaction is subjective. For example, a health professional may advise parents of the possibility of a mild reaction such as fever following immunisation. A fever may be the first occasion when their 8-week-old baby has been 'ill' and if the parents are also inexperienced, as most first-time parents are, such a reaction may be extremely worrying, especially if they are uncertain whether it might develop into something potentially more serious. Clearly, detailed information about what a parent can expect following immunisation will not remove the possibility of side-effects, but it may improve parents' coping abilities and thus reduce anxiety and, importantly, may make a parent feel more confident about returning for future immunisations.

In addition to the parents who wish to protect their child from the pain and distress associated with immunisation, there are those who express the belief that if their child were damaged, for example as a result of the pertussis vaccine, it would be entirely their fault, whereas if they caught natural whooping cough, it would be just that – natural, 'an act of God'. This belief was in spite of their awareness of the potential severity of the disease; it was perceived as something out of their control which was survivable. For these parents, advice from health professionals about the minimal risk attached to pertussis vaccine had not proved reassuring. One mother commented: 'Until they find a safe vaccine, 1:300,000 is still too large; I wouldn't play Russian roulette with my child'.[8]

Perceptions of immunisation as 'unnatural' and disease as 'natural', and in some cases beneficial, touch on the views of alternative practitioners which have been reviewed by Rogers and Pilgrim (unpublished).[4] The mother's comment on the risk of pertussis vaccine also raises questions about the usefulness of information for the general public that is based on risk assessment.

Information from the DoH and HEA generally takes a public health perspective, providing information supported by statistics, for example incidence of disease and risk of adverse events following immunisation. Much of this may be inappropriate for some parents, partly because it is irrelevant in the context of their concern for their own child who cannot be reduced to a statistic, but also because it is difficult to interpret. Many individuals are not familiar with risk assessment. The controversy surrounding whooping cough vaccine in the 1970s demonstrates the powerful effect of publicising a health risk associated with immunisation. Following publication of a paper suggesting a causal relationship between pertussis immunisation and serious neurological conditions,[12] there was a dramatic decline in acceptance of pertussis vaccine, followed by a large increase in cases of the disease. A large study called the National Childhood Encephalopathy Study (NCES) was set up to determine if the vaccine was associated with brain damage and, if so, to determine the size of the risk.[13] On the basis of the data collected it was concluded that the risk of a normal child developing permanent brain damage following whooping cough vaccine was 1 in 310,000.[14] Further studies have suggested that the risk may be even lower than suggested in the NCES. Acceptance of pertussis vaccine has gradually increased overall in this country and is now higher than 90%, but pertussis vaccine still causes anxiety for some parents[8,10] and health professionals.[6]

PARENTS' DIFFERING INFORMATION REQUIREMENTS

Research suggests that individual parents have differing information requirements.[15] A study commissioned by the HEA to provide guidance on the development of advertising gives useful insights into the possible variation of these requirements.[7] No information was given on the method of sample selection and the study is further limited by the small total sample size of 20 parents participating in either group discussions or interviews. Parents' attitudes fell into four categories; there is no indication what proportion of the parents were included in each category, but the total sample size inevitably means that some categories were very small. However, evidence from other studies supports the categorisation and it forms a useful basis for considering the needs of parents.

Automatic immunisers

Automatic immunisers tended to be first-time mothers who considered immunisation to be an automatic process which they did not question. They demonstrated little knowledge of side-effects apart from believing immunisation to be preferable to the risks of natural infection and showed little desire to investigate the issue of immunisation further. Health professionals were generally perceived to know best. Another study of 135 mothers of young children showed that for most of the mothers interviewed the decision to immunise had not been a problem: 'There was nothing to decide, I just knew I wanted them done'.[6]

Questioning immunisers

Questioning immunisers were more likely to have older children and they found the decision difficult, even the most difficult they had to make. They tended to worry more about the side-effects of immunisation, but ultimately decided to accept it. Such parents were also identified in Mayall and Grossmith's study and these parents had found the decision about pertussis vaccine in particular to be difficult.[9]

Elective immunisers/dissenters

This group represented parents who articulately expressed their views on the benefits and pitfalls of immunisation; they were extremely well informed and had either decided to accept or to reject immunisation. This was not an easy decision, they worried about it and often felt guilty, whatever their decision.

Selective immunisers

Parents in this category fell into two groups. There were those who were less influenced by their attitudes to immunisation and more by 'authorities' as a whole, such as parents who were fearful of being pinned down and, for example, losing social security benefits. The second group comprised parents who were living in temporary accommodation and were thus simply not in the right place at the right time to have their children immunised.

Parents may fall into different categories for different antigens. For example, a parent may be an automatic immuniser for diphtheria, tetanus, polio, Hib and MMR but a questioning immuniser for pertussis vaccine.

Information wanted by parents

There is considerable evidence that parents want more information about immunisation. The organisation The Informed Parent specifically sets out to provide information for parents and has a membership of over 1000. There is anecdotal evidence, from an author of this review (Helen Bedford) and other health professionals, that parents often request more detailed information and in particular papers from the scientific journals before they decide whether to accept immunisation.

Some studies have investigated the nature of information required by parents and the findings are reflected in the work of Gill and Sutton (1998)[3] who found that 42% of their sample wanted more information about immunisation. This included 45% (143) wanting to know more about side-effects and risks; 16% (50) exactly what each immunisation is and how it works; 15% (47) the diseases each immunisation protects against; 5% (15) about how much protection the immunisations provide; 3% (10) the risks of not immunising children; 2% (6) alternatives to immunisation; 1% (3) and information about the testing of immunisations, .

The information required by those individuals who reject immunisation is, as expected, more detailed. Rogers and Pilgrim (unpublished) found that these parents wanted information on alternatives to immunisation, the long- and short-term effects of immunisation, how the vaccines affect the immune system, and how the body copes with multiple vaccines.[4]

PARENTS WHO REJECT IMMUNISATION

In addition to the parents who decide not to complete a course of immunisation for their children, there is a small number of parents who decide from the outset that they do not wish their child to be immunised. Vaccine coverage figures represent completed courses and, as there are no national figures for consent rates, it is not clear what proportion of parents make this decision. However, some information is available from studies which suggests it is very small.

In Rogers and Pilgrim's study, only five of the 19 mothers decided at the outset not to accept immunisation.[4] Peckham *et al.* (1989) found that less than 1% of parents had refused consent to be included in the immunisation programme.[1] In Pearson *et al.*'s 1993 study[11] of 3585 children in Liverpool, 2% of parents had not consented to DT and polio, and 17% had refused consent for pertussis immunisation. In Bath District Health Authority, which has otherwise high immunisation rates, an investigation was conducted into the reasons why children received no immunisations. The prevalence of non-immunisation was 0.33% over the six-year period 1987–93.[16] It is likely that the proportion of parents rejecting immunisation varies both within and between districts. In a study conducted on behalf of the DoH, health visitors were surveyed by questionnaire in 21 districts.[17] Only 1 in 10 of respondents said that more than 3% of their clients rejected immunisation; these refusals were more likely in the low uptake districts, which were also more likely to be inner-city or urban districts. This supports the views of Ko *et al.* (1995) who point out that, although parents who reject immunisation are a small minority in their district, enabling the children of such parents to be immunised may be vital to reach national targets in areas where coverage is low.[18]

There is anecdotal evidence from practitioners that the number of parents who are choosing not to have their children immunised, although relatively few, is increasing[19] (*personal communication* – J. Moreton), although this needs to be investigated on a population basis. Paradoxically, this is not unexpected in view of the success of the immunisation programme and associated decline in infectious disease. Rogers and Pilgrim's study of rational non-compliance examined the issue in detail.[4] Their overall finding that a proportion of parents refuse immunisation because they consider it might be detrimental to their child's health is supported by Simpson's findings in 1995.[16] Part of this perception has developed from a belief in homeopathic treatment and from consulting alternative literature. Research at a national level is needed to quantify the amount of positive rejection among parents and to explore their reasons for this in depth. It is important to ensure that they are not basing their decision on misinformation.

HOMEOPATHY

There has been a considerable increase in interest surrounding alternative and complementary therapies in this country. For example, a survey in the UK in 1982 identified a total of 30,000 complementary practitioners of one sort or another. Subsequent developments have suggested a growth of 10% a year, making the present figure nearer 50,000.[20] A number of other surveys have shown the increasing use of complementary therapists by consumers and that an increasing number of GPs are enthusiastic about the benefits of homeopathy.[21–3] The Research Council for Complementary Medicine reported in 1996 that 1 in 10 people in Britain consult a practitioner of complementary medicine each year.[24] Some of the issues arising from the interest in homeopathy will be briefly considered here, since it is this branch of alternative medicine that has most relevance for immunisation uptake.

Homeopathy has been described as a system of treatment based on the principle that substances which cause symptoms can also be used to cure them. The homeopathic method attempts to match the symptoms of a sick person with the description of the toxic effects of a particular substance. The same substance in a much diluted form can then be safely used as a medicine or nosode.[25] In homeopathy there are no immunisations, but nosodes are given with the intention of increasing immunity. These are also used as a curative agent if an individual contracts disease. 'Pertussin 30' is the nosode given if there is a risk of contact with whooping cough. In the only published trial of the efficacy of 'pertussin 30', it was not possible to show that the vaccine was effective in preventing the disease.[26] It could be argued that the principles of conventional immunisation parallel the homeopathic method and it has been noted that Hahnemann, the physician who founded homeopathy, was a strong supporter of vaccination, considering it to be a clear and convincing demonstration of the Law of Similitude.[27]

Homeopaths' views on immunisation

Homeopathy is practised by practitioners with or without medical qualifications, and there is controversy among homeopathic practitioners about immunisation. In general, medically qualified practitioners, who are represented by the Faculty of Homeopathy, support immunisation and there is information to this effect included in the DoH memorandum (1996). Although the professional body of lay homeopaths, The Society of Homeopaths, does not have an official policy on immunisation, it considers that parents should have access to enough information to allow them to make an informed decision.[28] It has produced a leaflet entitled *Vaccination: a difficult decision* which, it has been argued: 'paints a highly tendentious and alarmist picture of immunisation, as well as containing some fundamental scientific errors'.[27]

In a paper which sought to provoke interest in homeopathy among doctors, Scott-Moncrieff (1991)[29] commented that, although homeopathy can be obtained on the NHS, resources are limited and individuals seeking treatment who are not prepared to wait for a long time often turn to the private sector. She points out that most private homeopathy is provided by lay practitioners who have a limited knowledge of pathology. This leaves them poorly placed to reach a correct diagnosis and to make referrals to more appropriate practitioners if necessary. In addition, she considers that they often have highly unscientific ideas about health care and, using immunisation as a particular example, comments that once parents have been told they are harming their children by allowing them to be immunised, it is exceedingly difficult to persuade them otherwise.[29]

A considerable amount of literature puts forward the lay homeopathic position on immunisation: it is generally opposed to immunisation. The major issues have been considered by Rogers and Pilgrim (unpublished).[4] Although Fisher (1990)[27] believes that the anti-immunisation lobby has the right to debate its case, he argues that it 'must not be permitted to hitch its wagon to homeopathy's rising star'. In his paper Fisher considers the writings of Harris Coulter in particular, who has written widely on the subject of mass immunisation and links a variety of problems with it including criminality, a reduction in the IQ of American children, and sudden infant death syndrome.[30] Fisher believes that few of his arguments are sound but also points out that: 'it is possible that immunisation has insidious low grade chronic effects which have not yet been detected' but that the abandonment of mass immunisation, which is in effect what Coulter recommends, would be 'criminally irresponsible'.

Implications for health professionals

In a brief review of two of the main sources of anti-immunisation literature, Elliman (1993)[19] points out that Chaitow (1988)[31] and Coulter (1991)[30] use material from mainstream scientific literature which has been either selectively chosen or misquoted to illustrate a particular point. By presenting individual accounts of children purported to be vaccine-damaged, they provide highly emotive material which is often quoted as though it were a scientific source. The use of selective quotes or misquotes from the mainstream literature to support their extreme views enables Chaitow and Coulter to construct powerful arguments which appear to have scientific validity and would add fuel to the views of any individual who had doubts about immunisation. Many parents may be keen to explore all avenues before deciding whether to accept immunisation, but those who do not have a scientific background may not be able to subject such views to analytical scrutiny and may need the guidance of health professionals in unravelling the issues.

Rogers and Pilgrim found that a number of parents in their study had given alternative literature to their GP or health visitor in order to facilitate a discussion.[4] The responses to this were varied but generally non-responsive, and in one case a GP de-registered the child a few weeks after the mother had given her a copy of Chaitow's book.

Elliman (1993) believes health professionals need to be aware of the anti-immunisation literature, to be armed with a good knowledge of the present-day status of immunisation and infectious diseases, and to be prepared to discuss the issues raised in the literature in detail.[19] Practising health professionals are not always well equipped to do this and, as a particular letter to a professional journal demonstrates, can be equally susceptible to the arguments forwarded by the anti-immunisation lobby.[32] Elliman has produced a detailed critique of Chaitow's work for distribution to individual parents in his district. This type of information is urgently required for more general circulation to both health professionals and parents.

SUMMARY

- Parents' attitudes to immunisation are very important and are shaped by a wide interplay of influences. These, together with past experience of immunisation, may have more influence on a parent's decision about immunisation than the empirical advice from health professionals alone. However, there is still considerable scope to improve communication skills and information giving.

- Bad experiences related to immunisation may prevent not only future acceptance of immunisation but also take up of other primary health care services.

- Vaccine reactions are a major cause of worry for parents even though these may appear to be mild to health professionals. Parents need to be given detailed and accurate advice about the nature and likelihood of side-effects and about methods of treatment, together with information about who they should contact if they are concerned.

- There is a small but increasing number of individuals and groups who are opposed to or have serious criticisms about immunisation. As immunisation rates continue to improve they will assume greater importance as a group who may need targeting. While it is every parent's right to make an informed choice not to have their child immunised, it is important to ensure that this decision is not based on misinformation.

- Much of the literature produced by groups and individuals who are opposed to or have serious criticisms about immunisation is unscientific and relies on anecdote to increase fears about the safety and efficacy of immunisation.

Health professionals need to be familiar with the literature and be prepared to take time to discuss the issues raised in detail with those parents who seek such discussion.

- There is considerable scope for professionals to improve their communication skills in both information giving and eliciting and responding to parents' beliefs and fears.

- Parents want more information about immunisation and have differing information requirements. For example, parents who consult the alternative literature require information which specifically focuses on the issues it raises. There is a need to investigate precise and differing information requirements in greater detail.

References

1. Peckham, C., Bedford, H., Senturia, Y., Ades, A. *National Immunisation Study: factors influencing immunisation uptake in childhood*. 1989. Action Research, Horsham.

2. Christie, A.B. 'Measles', in *Infectious diseases: epidemiology and clinical practice*. 1980. Churchill Livingstone, Edinburgh.

3. Gill, E., Sutton, S. 'Immunisation uptake: the role of parental attitudes' in Hey, V. (ed.) *Immunisation research: a summary volume*. 1998. HEA, London.

4. Rogers, A., Pilgrim, D. 'Non-compliance with childhood immunisation: personal accounts of parents and health care professionals' Unpublished.

5. Senior, M.L., New, S.J., Gatrell, A.C., Francis, B.J. 'Geographic influences on the uptake of infant immunisations: 1. Concepts, models and aggregate analyses', *Environment and Planning A*, 1993; 25: 425–36.

6. Mayall, B., Foster, M.C. *Child health care: living with children, working for children*. 1989. Heinemann Nursing, Oxford.

7. Health Education Authority. 'Childhood immunisation advertising campaign'. 1993. Unpublished report for the HEA, London.

8. New, S.J., Senior, M.L. '"I don't believe in needles": qualitative aspects of a study into the uptake of infant immunisation in two English health authorities', *Social Science & Medicine*, 1991; 33(4): 509–18.

9. Mayall, B., Grossmith, C. 'Using preventive child health services', *Health Visitor*, 1985; 58: 293–5.

10. Bennett, P., Smith, C. 'Parents' attitudes towards immunisation in Wales according to socio-economic group: a preliminary investigation', *Health Education Journal*, 1992; 51(3): 127–31.

11. Pearson, M., Makowiecka, K., Gregg, J., Woollard, J., Rogers, M., West, C. 'Primary immunisation in Liverpool, I: who withholds consent?' *Archives of Disease in Childhood*, 1993; 69: 110–14.

12. Kulenkampff, M., Schwartzmen, J.S., Wilson, J. 'Neurological complications of pertussis inoculation.' *Archives of Disease in Childhood*,1974; (49): 46–9.

13. Miller, D., Ross, E.M., Alderslade, R., Bellman, M.H., Rawson, N.S.B. 'Pertussis immunisation and serious acute neurological illnesses in children', *British Medical Journal*, 1981; 282: 1595–9.

14. Committee on Safety of Medicines and The Joint Committee on Vaccination and Immunisation. *Whooping cough*. 1984. HMSO, London.

15. Fitzgerald, T.M., Glotzer, D.E. 'Vaccine information pamphlets: more information than parents want?', *Pediatrics*, 1995; 95(3) 331–4.

16. Simpson, N., Lenton, S., Randall, R. 'Parental refusal to have children immunised: extent and reasons', *British Medical Journal*, 1995; 310: 227.

17. British Market Research Bureau. *The uptake of pre-school immunisation in England*. 1989. BMRB.

18. Ko, M.L.B., Rao, M., Taere, L., Bridgman, G.C.B., Kurian, A. 'Outcome of referrals to a district immunisation advisory clinic', *Communicable Disease Report*, 1995; 5(10): R146–R149.

19. Elliman, D. 'The doubter's bookshelf', *Newsletter of British Association for Community Child Health (BACCH)*, 1993.

20. Pietroni, P.C. 'Beyond the boundaries: relationship between general practice and complementary medicine', in Pringle, M. (ed.) *Change and teamwork in primary care*. 1993. British Medical Journal, London.

21. Unauthored. 'Magic or medicine?', *Which?* 1981.

22. Unauthored. 'Mori poll', *The Times*, 1989; 13 November.

23. Unauthored. 'GP thumbs up for homeopathy', *Doctor*, 1992; 16 July.

24. Goldbeck-Wood, S. 'Complementary medicine is booming worldwide', *British Medical Journal*, 1996; 313: 131–3.

25. Gemmell, D.M. *Everyday homeopathy*. 1987. Beaconsfield Publishers Ltd, Beaconsfield.

26. English, J.M. 'Pertussin 30 – preventive for whooping cough?', *The British Homeopathic Journal*, 1987; 76: 61–5.

27. Fisher, P. 'Enough nonsense on immunisation', *The British Homeopathic Journal*, 1990; 79: 198–200.

28. Lee, F. 'Letter to the editor', *The British Homeopathic Journal*, 1991; 80: 70–1.

29. Scott-Moncrieff, C. 'Contract gives boost to GP homeopathy', *Pulse*, 1991; 12 January.

30. Coulter, H.L., Fisher, B.L. *A shot in the dark*. 1991. Avery, New York.

31. Chaitow, L. *Vaccination and immunisation: dangers, delusions and alternatives*. 1988. C.W. Daniel Company, Saffron Walden.

32. O'Connell, D. 'Against immunisation' (letter), *Health Visitor*, 1993; 66: 225.

6. Consumers' views of the child health services with particular reference to immunisation

Ideally, the evaluation of any professional practice should address itself to those who are receiving and allegedly benefiting from the service. However, much of the practice in relation to the child health service, especially health visiting, is carried out in a 'private' capacity and the views of the consumer have rarely been sought.[1] Thus, little is known about what actually occurs between a practitioner and client and what the client's views are in terms of the effectiveness of the service.

In this section, the available literature on client perceptions and satisfaction with the child health service will be reviewed. The focus will be on health visiting, as this group have traditionally been largely responsible for talking to parents about immunisation.

Graham's 1979 study of women's views of the child health service was one of the first to question the structure and organisation of the child health services from the client's point of view.[2] She found that levels of satisfaction with the child health services and the health visitor declined with increasing age of the child: 70% of mothers had positive perceptions at one month post-partum and 56% at five months, although it also should be borne in mind that contacts with the health visitor decrease over time. The functions mothers attributed to the health visitor included checking on weight, advising on problems, and enhancing social life, and health visitors performed these functions satisfactorily. Although Graham does not comment on the positive perceptions of the health visitor's role, she attributes the negative comments (44% after five months) to a negative perception of the health visitor's role – as one of inspecting or policing. Another factor which appeared to be important in the rejection of child health services was a previous experience in the clinic, for example, which had caused humiliation to the mother or made her feel inadequate. Graham's survey does not reveal further factors which may be associated with a rejection of the health visiting service, such as the individual communication skills used by the health visitor.[2]

The influence of previous negative experiences as a factor in non-acceptance or incompletion of immunisation has been discussed. Rogers and Pilgrim's insights[3] into negative experiences have implications for the way in which parents are received in the child health clinic and the degree to which promotion of immunisation is seen as propaganda. Graham's observations support those of Rogers and Pilgrim that negative perceptions surrounding immunisation may also have an impact on the uptake of other child health services, including child health surveillance and use of primary health care services in general.

A study of parents' perceptions of the child health clinic has indicated that, whilst over half the respondents appreciated the reassurance and advice of the health visitor, there was a need to provide more privacy and a play area in the clinic.[4] It is not possible to describe parents' views about immunisation specifically from this study, but there is an implication that an improved clinic environment might further encourage parents to attend for the child health services, including immunisation.

Field *et al.* (1982) interviewed women about their views on the health visiting service and also found 60% (78) of the sample were positive, but again no clear suggestions are made about perceptions of the role of health visitors from the positive commentators.[5] Among the 40% who made negative comments, the findings were similar to Graham's, revealing factors such as authoritarianism, a perceived interfering attitude, and lack of sympathy. In addition, childless health visitors were not seen as useful, although there is little elaboration on this.

Moss *et al.* (1986)[6] studied mothers at six months post-partum and found, like Graham, that socio-economic group becomes an important factor in attitudes to services at around the six-month period when clients of socio-economic groups IV and V become increasingly dissatisfied with health visitors. They speculate that this could be due to the social distance which often exists between the health visitor and the more socio-economically deprived clients, and also because such women had a wide kinship network in the vicinity and the help of relatives was valued more than that of the health visitor.

Orr's 1980 study of socio-economically deprived women in Ulster remains one of the few in-depth studies of health visiting, and also highlights clients' perceptions of the need for health visitors in the early months of motherhood.[7] This retrospective survey of 68 women found that health visitors were generally held in a favourable light and that home visiting was an acceptable activity to over two-thirds of the sample. However, dissatisfaction was expressed with fragmentation of services, poor clinic facilities which prevented private conversation with health visitors, a tendency by health visitors to call unannounced, and a need for health visitors to improve their interpersonal skills. Orr's study is very valuable since it has addressed the needs and perceptions of a minority group – socio-economically deprived Ulster women. However, it has limitations since it was a retrospective survey and thereby relied on the women's memory of their interactions. There may be a problem with validity – the women may have been reflecting their mood on the day of the interview onto health visitors. It presents only the women's views: health visitors were not given an opportunity to give their side of the story and there is no material which supports the women's evidence regarding the interpersonal skills of the health visitors.

MODELS OF HEALTH VISITING

A more recent survey by Foster and Mayall (1990), however, has produced similar findings.[8] In their study of views of child health services among 33 mothers with a first child of 21 months, the views of parents in an inner-city area were compared with those of a randomised group in the suburbs of London. The study was based on a longitudinal design so that parents were interviewed three times over a period of one year to reach an understanding of their perspectives of the preventive child health services over time. Unlike Orr (1980),[7] the researchers in this study used open-ended, in-depth interviewing and they also interviewed the health visitors involved with the families. The study suggests that, from the health visitors' perspective, a behavioural model of education is adopted which the authors describe as authoritarian and pedagogical. This would support one of the styles described by Rogers and Pilgrim (unpublished) – the 'authoritarian' position – on the basis of their interviews with GPs and health visitors.[3]

Foster and Mayall (1990) found that, even when health visitors rejected an authoritarian style, they favoured a model of health education which assumed the health visitor was the expert and knew what kind of behaviour would be 'best' for the client.[8] This may be seen as a more paternalistic approach as also described by Rogers and Pilgrim (unpublished)[3] and McKinstry (1992).[9]

In contrast, the clients in Foster and Mayall's (1990) study generally disapproved of the 'top down' approach and felt that their own expertise in childcare was undermined by the health visitor's introduction of topics regardless of the mother's knowledge.[8] Mothers felt discouraged from bringing up particular issues if they did not like the approach of the health visitor. They cite one example which has particular relevance: a mother had wanted detailed information about immunisation because of a family history of convulsions but found it difficult to talk to the health visitor because her manner was patronising.

The mothers in Foster and Mayall's study liked the health visitors who adopted a partnership approach in their dialogue.[8] The authors largely explain their findings in terms of educational theory – that the education of health visitors is inadequate, leading to practitioners who are limited in their ability to create meaningful dialogue but instead adopt a 'top down' or interventionist approach. Whilst recognising the importance of one-to-one interaction, Foster and Mayall go on to recommend a *community action approach* to health visiting as proposed by Drennan (1985).[10] It appears that their evidence for the need for this approach comes not directly from the clients in the study but from the sociological literature.[11] Although Drennan's work was encouraging in that it suggested a new direction for health visiting, it must be acknowledged that health visitors may not yet have either the philosophy or the skills appropriate for working effectively with community groups whose needs may be complex. In particular, this would be a radical departure in the immunisation debate.

The main indication of the studies reviewed so far is that clients welcome home visits as long as the health visitors are 'friendly', non-judgmental, and sensitive to the needs as the client sees them, whilst accepting that the client does have expertise in child-rearing.

Two further studies have looked in more depth at the interpersonal skills exercised by health visitors as experienced by the clients. Ashley (1987) took a feminist approach to explain women's experience of health visitors and interpretation of their needs.[12] The study focused on the needs of 28 women, as interpreted by themselves, attending one of three women's groups. Ashley found, like previous researchers,[7] that women perceived their health visitors in a friendly light but misconceived their role as far as their own problems were concerned. The women in the study were more likely to understand the health visitors' function in terms of childcare rather than in terms of their own health, especially their mental health.[12] Ashley suggests that this reluctance to discuss emotional problems with the health visitor is largely because health visitors portray themselves as professionals who are only interested in childcare and mothering, again perhaps a reflection of the paternalistic approach.[12]

The women in this study had rejected mother and toddler groups because they felt that the inadequacies they were experiencing would be on public display. This also reflects findings that some parents feel inadequate when attending the child health clinic, where there is a perceived pressure to immunise children when they have made a positive decision not to.[3] Ashley infers that health visitors do not recognise the desire among women for their needs to be met through a community action model. However, the fact that these women were attending self-help groups implies that they were particularly self-motivated, similar in many respects to Rogers and Pilgrim's sample.[3] Like other researchers,[8] Ashley suggests that health visitors should approach their aims of facilitating health-enhancing activities through a *community model* rather than the *individualised developmental model*. However, although Ashley found support for the 'friendly' approach of some health visitors, she does not address the skills that health visitors would need to acquire in order to work in the community in this way.[12]

Foxman *et al.* (1982) interviewed 96 women six weeks post-partum to elicit their response to the health visiting service.[13] Although the majority (61%) were positive towards their health visitor, negative comments were mostly made in relation to interpersonal skills and the authors conclude that: 'our findings underline the importance of communication skills which can help health visitors tailor their responses to the needs of individual mothers'. Although Foxman *et al.* suggest further research in this area, they do not elaborate on the nature of the skills or the research they propose.

An unpublished paper[14] demonstrated the complexities of working with vulnerable groups in the community. This project looked at health visitors working with prostitutes in AIDS prevention and highlights the high level of interpersonal skills that are required to maintain meaningful dialogue and reach an understanding of role between the health visitor and client. One skill in particular, which health visitors in other studies have not demonstrated, was flexibility. For example, McIntosh's qualitative study of interpersonal skills in health visiting in 1986 revealed a very rigid approach as perceived by the clients.[15] The findings of this study were based on six semi-structured interviews carried out among 60 women from lower socio-economic groups from the seventh month of pregnancy until the ninth month of the baby's life. McIntosh suggests that the 'professional style of the health visitor was ... central to the establishment of an effective rapport with mothers'. Thus the health visitors who used a *relationship-centred approach* were more likely to be effective in terms of client action than those adopting a *problem-orientated approach*.[15] However, McIntosh is not able to qualify this judgment and, like Ashley and others, relies on the client's report of the health visitor's style rather than direct evidence.

McIntosh also found a high degree of unmet need among his sample of 60 socio-economically deprived women.[15] Mental and emotional problems amongst the women were common, as was the need for practical assistance. Often these problems were interrelated. For example, a persistently crying baby led to some mothers feeling angry and isolated and they felt that somewhere to take the child occasionally would be helpful. Health visitors were not perceived as playing a helpful role in this type of problem because they were seen as being judgmental of the mother's competence and were associated with aspects of social control, including the detection of child abuse and neglect. Immunisation has to be viewed within the context of health for the whole family and, clearly, there are implications here for the likelihood of parents taking up immunisation under these conditions. McIntosh largely accounts for the generally negative attitudes expressed towards the health visitors by the nature of the interpersonal skills: 'The health visitor's personality, approach and interpersonal skills are of paramount importance in determining her degree of acceptability'.[15]

However, other studies[2,7,13] have not produced such negative findings as McIntosh and this can perhaps be explained by timing. Some studies have interviewed mothers early in their experience of motherhood, whilst McIntosh's sample were interviewed throughout pregnancy and well into the first year of life. It is recognised by McIntosh and others that clients are more positive towards the child health services in the early weeks of parenthood. Also, McIntosh's sample is unusual in that all the women were socio-economically deprived and came from a culture (Glasgow) which traditionally has strong kinship networks, suggesting that the women do not feel the need for 'outside' help as much as others. However, despite these anomalies, McIntosh's study is an important contribution to the understanding of the effectiveness of health visiting through the client's eyes. McIntosh concludes by recognising the need for an *egalitarian model* of health visiting: 'Giving choice to the consumer, over what help to seek and when, implies a more equal and participating relationship between client and professional'.[15] The implication of the study, like others, is that health visiting should be a *responsive* service, not an *interventionist* activity.

THE 'INTERMEDIATE DOMAIN'

Mayall (1993) has attempted to explain some of the difficulties encountered by mothers and health visitors in terms of an 'intermediate domain'.[16] This is based on an analysis of two previous studies which suggest that the gendered nature of childcare implies that women are both the paid and unpaid carers of child health. This makes negotiations difficult in the sense that, whilst both parties accept the overall need for a state concern in child welfare, there is continuous refining of each other's part in childcare work and each other's knowledge. Mayall suggests that: 'The acceptance by women of caring as women's work allows them to cross boundaries between the private and public domains to create and delineate an intermediate domain where acceptance of each others' abilities is recognised and contributions made'.[16]

The most difficult aspects of these negotiations are where public policies conflict with private childcare practices and neither the health visitor nor the mother are in a position to challenge the social policy framework. As health visitors effectively feel powerless to enable the mother to provide good care in the context of poverty, for example, they feel tension between their loyalty to the mother and to the state. How far they decide to extend their advocacy role on behalf of the mother or to carry out their obligations to the state may account for some of the 'sharp disagreement, antagonism and suspicion' described by Mayall (1993)[16] and revealed by others using different conceptual frameworks.

THE PURPOSE OF THE HOME VISIT

A survey by Watson and Sim (1989) involved the exploration of mothers' and health visitors' perceptions of home visits in an inner-city area.[17] A sample of 100 health visitors and clients were interviewed following a home visit to ascertain their perceptions of the purpose of the visit. Watson and Sim found that, in general, health visitors and clients agreed on the visit contents.

In contrast, Kendall's (1991) study of 75 home visits by health visitors found a low level of agreement between health visitors and mothers about their perceptions of the visit.[18] Mothers and health visitors were interviewed independently following a home visit along four dimensions – the perceived purpose of the visit, perceptions of health need, perceptions of intended action, and perceptions of follow-up. In relation to immunisation, 28% (21) of the health visitors perceived this to be part of the purpose of the visit, whilst none of the mothers mentioned immunisation as part of the purpose. This is of concern because parents cannot prepare their questions or express their anxieties if they are not aware that immunisation is on the agenda, a situation that will be particularly true at the new birth visit. Interestingly, in relation to the perceived plan of action, 9.3% (7) of the clients perceived immunisation to be part of the plan, compared to 18.7% (14) of the health visitors. This suggests two things. First, although immunisation was not on the perceived agenda, a small number of mothers were nevertheless prepared to take action. Secondly, there were a similar number of mothers who did not perceive this as part of their intended action, despite the health visitor's belief that it was. This type of dissonance, although not significant, may indicate that health visitors and other primary health care practitioners should clarify with their clients what their objectives are, and provides further support for the suggestion that a chance to prepare questions may improve intentions to take up immunisation.

This difference in findings between Kendall's study[18] and Watson and Sim's study[17] may be explained by the large sample in the latter study who came from non-English-speaking backgrounds – 38% were Bengali. Not only did this necessitate the use of translators in some cases, which may have distorted the findings, but culturally, Bengali women are much more likely to be compliant with perceived representatives of authority. This is substantiated by Watson and Sim's finding that 100% of the Bengali women had found the visit helpful and 82% wanted more visits, compared with only 18% of other women in the study. An additional criticism of Watson and Sim's study is that a very quantitative approach was taken to the interviews which may have led to mothers being unable to discuss important issues. Perhaps most significantly, whilst the authors draw inferences about the level of agreement between health visitor and client during a home visit, they cannot substantiate this with any observational or interaction data. Kendall's work, on the other hand, was corroborated by detailed analysis of the health visitor–client interaction.

EMPOWERING PARENTS

Vehvilainen-Julkenen (1993) found that, following preparation for parenthood classes using an empowering approach, 80 mothers and fathers who completed a questionnaire expressed feelings of competence and control in their lives six months after the classes.[19] The parents identified the key practitioners as the midwife, the public health nurse, other parents in the group and the physician. The main focus of the intervention was small group work. This *empowerment approach* seems to be highly regarded by the clients in this study, but takes the position which Rogers and Pilgrim (unpublished) describe as 'liberal paternalistic'.[3] This implies that the profession will accept the client's decision, which may be not to immunise.

SUMMARY

- Parents value the health visiting service most in the early months of parenthood.

- A socio-economic group distinction is apparent in satisfaction with health visitors.

- Much of the dissatisfaction is centred around interpersonal skills and role perceptions.

- There is scope for developing more participative approaches to child health issues, such as community work or small group work.

References

1. Mayall, B., Foster, M.C. *Parents and health visitors: perspectives on preventive health care.* 1988. Thomas Coram Research Unit, London.

2. Graham, H. 'Women's attitudes to the child health services', *Health Visitor*, 1979; 52: 175–8.

3. Rogers, A., Pilgrim, D. 'Non-compliance with childhood immunisation: personal accounts of parents and health care professionals' Unpublished.

4. Sefi, S., Grice, D. 'Parents' views of clinics', *Health Visitor*, 1994; 67(20): 62.

5. Field, S., Draper, J., Kerr, M., Hare, M. 'A consumer view of the health visiting service', *Health Visitor*, 1982; 55(6): 299–301.

6. Moss, O., Bollard, G., Foxman, R., Owen, C. 'The first six months after birth: mother's views and health visitors', *Health Visitor*, 1986; 59(3): 71–4.

7. Orr, J. *Health visiting in focus.* 1980. Royal College of Nursing, London.

8. Foster, M.C., Mayall, B. 'Health visitors as educators', *Journal of Advanced Nursing*, 1990; 15: 286–92.

9. McKinstry, B. 'Paternalism and the doctor–patient relationship in general practice', *British Journal of General Practice*, 1992; 42: 340–2.

10. Drennan, V. *Working in a different way.* 1985. North Paddington District Health Authority, London.

11. Friere, P. *Pedagogy of the oppressed.* 1972. Penguin, Harmondsworth.

12. Ashley, Y. 'Do health visitors really understand women's health needs?' 1987. *Proceedings of the International Primary Health Care Conference.*

13. Foxman, R., Moss, P., Bolard, G., Owen, C. 'A consumer view of the health visitor at six weeks post-partum', *Health Visitor*, 1982; 55(6): 302–8.

14. Thomson, A. Unpublished paper given at the *Nursing Times* Primary Health Care Conference. November 1988.

15. McIntosh, J. *A consumer perspective on the health visiting service*. 1986. Social and Paediatric Research Unit, University of Glasgow.

16. Mayall, B. 'Keeping children healthy - the intermediate domain', *Social Science & Medicine*, 1993; 36(1): 77–83.

17. Watson, E., Sim, J. 'The health visitor's visit', *Health Visitor*, 1989; 62(7): 214–17.

18. Kendall, S. 'The influence of the health visiting process on client participation: an analysis of the health visitor–client interaction'. 1991. Unpublished Ph.D. thesis, King's College London.

19. Vehvilainen-Julkenen, K. 'Empowering clients in parenthood education', *Journal of Clinical Nursing*, 1993; 2(4): 256–9.

7. Professional–client interaction studies

This section reviews literature related to the interaction between health professional and client, selected on the basis of the quality of the research and its relevance to primary health care and specifically to immunisation. Inevitably, there are a number of health visiting studies worthy of attention and some studies conducted in the paediatric setting have been included. A number of studies from medicine and social work have informed and influenced research into the qualitative aspects of primary health care interactions with clients, so some of these are also included.

Within the vast literature on communication there exist many methodologies, both quantitative and qualitative, for analysing interactions. For example, a review of 61 studies found 28 different analytical techniques.[1] It is therefore not appropriate to carry out a formal meta-analysis of these studies and a narrative account of the studies will be presented, drawing out the implications for the immunisation aspects of a consultation.

Twenty-two years after Johnson and Hardin's (1962) study of public health nursing,[2] Clark (1984) described audio recording as a method of collecting data on the health visitor–client interaction.[3] Although the method had been used in studies of related disciplines,[4-7] Clark suggested that the study of the health visitor–client interaction posed special problems as 'the talk which is exchanged between the health visitor and client, especially during home visits, is relatively unfocused and unstructured'.[3]

Baldock and Prior (1981) previously reported an analysis of conversations between social workers and clients in which they suggested that the interviews were often unstructured, with a 'curiously ramshackle air'.[5] This implies that the health visiting interview was not unique in its style, and was amenable to analytical approaches demonstrated by research in related areas which would shed new light on the nature of health visiting practice.

CLIENT-CENTRED APPROACHES

Byrne and Long's (1976) study of the talk occurring between doctors and patients had considerable influence on subsequent studies.[4] They analysed the interactions occurring in over 2500 medical consultations in general practice and developed a scoring system for rating the interactions according to six identified phases of the interview: relating to the patient, discovering the reason for the patient's attendance, conducting verbal or physical examination or both, consideration of patient condition, treatment or investigation, and termination.

Within each of these phases interactional styles were identified, for example clarifying and direct questioning, and the styles were numbered from 1 to 7 across a continuum of doctor-centredness (1) to patient-centredness (7). This categorisation was then used to score the interaction and used as an indicator of the doctor's overall style. The study revealed that the doctors generally tended towards a doctor-centred approach and the authors attributed this largely to the medical model of education and other factors such as short consultation time in busy city practices. However, an inherent problem which arises from this study is the scoring system, which depended on raters identifying the style and assigning it the appropriate style number. A style which fell between two styles was assigned a fractional score (e.g. 2½). The lack of information regarding the reliability of this rather arbitrary scoring system suggests that it is not necessarily a useful instrument for studying professional–client interaction in other disciplines.

Although Baldock and Prior (1981)[5] used the Byrne and Long analytical technique described above, they give very little attention to their analytical framework and it is therefore difficult to make an objective assessment of the conclusions they reach about social work interviews. They suggest that social workers are more client-centred than doctors and yet use controlling mechanisms in a latent fashion, which Baldock and Prior argue is skilled practice. The work has been criticised on the grounds that a non-directive approach which leaves the client 'confused, and indeed deceived'[8] cannot be described as skilled if the skills are not in line with the meaning that clients assigned to social work help.

This criticism has implications for the current review – can immunisation be promoted without some understanding of the client's interpretation of events or their perception of the activities of the primary health care team?

INFORMED DECISION MAKING

Tuckett *et al.* (1982) addressed this issue when they investigated the GP–patient interaction in terms of the integration of lay and medical frameworks of knowledge during an educational exchange.[9] The objective was one of exploring informed decision making among patients in general practice and the analysis was based on 405 audio-recorded consultations and subsequent interviewing of a sample of 328 patients at home. The research was rigorous in its analytical framework and reliability testing and the conclusions have considerable bearing on the current review. Although Tuckett and colleagues identified nine positive elements of the consultations (e.g. patients could generally correctly interpret the meaning of important points made about their condition), they also identified 11 negative elements (e.g. an absence of reactive justification, that is, doctors justifying their action in response to patient cues on demand), which led them to conclude that overall, 'consultations are not enabling patients to make informed decisions about their health care, and are not being conducted to use this interactive potential'.[9]

This clearly has implications for the way in which the immunisation discussion develops between the health professional and the client, since the decision being made is not simply the client's decision but a decision being made on behalf of the child. It is particularly important for the parents that their decisions are as informed as possible.

INDIVIDUAL FACTORS

Roter *et al.*'s 1988 review of 61 interaction studies drew some useful generalisations including the finding that whites received more information than other ethnic groups and that there is probably a tendency for patients from higher socio-economic groups to ask more questions than patients from lower socio-economic groups.[1] Roter and colleagues criticise researchers for not documenting variables such as socio-economic group, race and age carefully in this type of research, thus making it difficult to draw firm conclusions. However, the review itself is conducted rigorously with sound quality-control mechanisms making it likely that the indications above are valid. It is therefore relevant to bear these points in mind when considering the implications for practice in the immunisation context and this would appear to bear out some of the findings mentioned in the section above on consumer views. The professional–client interaction studies described previously raise the question that, if the health visitor, 'by promoting health and health policies, empowers people to take responsibility for health as individuals, families and communities, and thereby helps to prevent and minimise the effects of disease, dysfunction and disability',[10] to what extent is she/he using the potential of the interaction to achieve this?

NEGOTIATION OF GOALS

Previous studies of the relationship between health visitors and clients have reached different conclusions. Warner (1984) conducted a study of the interaction between health visitors and clients in the clinic situation by capturing audio-recorded data of 229 interactions.[11] She expressed her interest as being centred around the 'ways in which practitioners fit advice to individual clients' and was more interested in the dynamic aspect of the interaction than in content.

This study is different from other studies of health visiting by virtue of the contextual issues. Clearly, the clinic is a very different situation from the home visit; in the clinic health visitors are playing a responsive role in that the client comes to them. Visits to the clinic are more public than visits in the home; others may overhear details of childcare practices and advice given by the health visitor. Thus, the clinic consultation is more akin to the medical consultation in that the interview is usually limited in time, the client attends for a specific purpose which may be known to both health visitor and client, and there is likely to be a public element such as a waiting room and a receptionist which may have a bearing on who attends the clinic and what they are prepared to divulge.

Warner gives examples from her analysis of how health visitors use interactional techniques to both encourage clients to ask the 'right' questions and to move towards mutually achieved goals.[11] The techniques she describes include offering the mother objective evidence, diminishing the mother's responsibility for an observed problem, and building on the mother's existing knowledge and practice. In much the same way as Baldock and Prior (1981) described the hidden techniques that social workers use to control their clients,[5] Warner suggests that health visitors pursue their plans with 'remarkable tenacity' and her descriptions of interactions indicate that the techniques used by the health visitors were covert. The author concludes that plans were 'interactionally achieved during encounters as the health visitor modified her plan minute by minute to suit the client's readiness to co-operate with the plan.[11]

The overall impression gained from this study is that, although Warner perceives the goals to be 'mutually acceptable' and achieved by 'negotiation', there is little evidence for goals being openly negotiated, and a lack of client follow-up in the study leaves room for more speculation as far as the client's perception of the goals is concerned. As the child health clinic is a major route by which immunisation is discussed and taken up, it would seem appropriate to negotiate goals and actions more overtly.

Health promotion talk between doctors and patients has been described and it is again evident that the professional and client rarely share a frame of reference. In one study, 200 tape-recorded encounters between doctors and patients in a primary health care setting were analysed. The difficulty observed in doctors and patients sharing health promotion talk may imply that health professionals have to consider this as a special conversational task in order to be effective.[12]

An early study of doctor–parent communication in the paediatric setting arrived at some interesting findings.[13] Statistical analysis of 38 interactions revealed that paediatricians talked for twice as long, and proportionally asked twice as many questions and gave twice as many commands as did the parents. One explanation for this is that there is not enough time in the encounter to negotiate role relationships. While this study was published in 1982, the constraints on time in the interaction are still very relevant and it must be worth considering how the time spent with parents can be most effectively utilised.

Negotiation and setting of goals with parents in relation to immunisation must be seen as high priority within the limited time available to health professionals. In support of this, a study of 115 paediatrician–parent interactions found that parents who were more able to ask questions and express concerns received more information from the physician. The sample consisted of 86% white parents and the majority were educated at least to college level. However, whilst the author acknowledges the importance of education, it is also suggested that health professionals should pay attention to *clients' communicative styles*.[14]

INTERACTIONAL STYLES

Sefi (1985) carried out a detailed study of health visiting in order to 'find out what occurs between the health visitor and mother during a routine visit in the mother's home'.[15] She collected audio recordings of all visits to ten new mothers by five health visitors from birth of the baby to 8 weeks. From a total of 46 tapes, nine tapes relating to the primary visit (i.e. ten days postnatally) were selected for transcription and analysis. Sefi posed three main research questions:

- What is the extent to which the interaction consists of advice giving or support?

- Is the nature of the interaction professional/client in orientation or one of befriending?

- What kind of strategies are used in the giving of advice?[15]

As far as is known, neither health visitors nor clients were 'primed' prior to the interactions being recorded. Sefi subjected her data to both quantitative and qualitative analysis. The quantitative analysis revealed that health visitors spent proportionally more time on baby-orientated topics than mother-orientated topics and they opened and closed all topics. This tends to suggest a controlling aspect of style directed more at problems than relationship building. However, the small sample in this study must be acknowledged.

Sefi took an ethnomethodological approach to the qualitative analysis and turns to conversation analysis (as described in Heritage, 1984)[16] for her analytical framework. Although the transcriptions were carefully carried out according to the notation of the school of conversation analysis, Montgomery-Robinson (1987)[17] has criticised Sefi on the grounds that she does not make it clear where she wishes her study to stand methodologically. The analysis was validated by a second researcher (John Heritage).

Sefi did, in fact, make some detailed observations on the structure of the health visitor–client interaction but it is arguable whether conversation analysis *per se*, which as Sefi takes pains to point out is a costly and time-consuming process, was the only method appropriate for analysing these data. For example, Sefi identified the 'question/answer/third-turn sequence' as a construct of health visitor–client talk. She identified that the third turn 'overwhelmingly consists of the health visitor delivering either advice or information or endorsement'. She analysed this third turn in terms of it being either authoritative or affiliative and concluded that, in general, it tended to be authoritative. Sefi asserts that health visitors get through all their business via this technique. She concluded that the health visitor maintains a controlling influence over the interaction with clients and that, 'In general, the consequences of the assertion of professional knowledge was to cast the mother in the role of the uninformed recipient of information and as a person whose competence in the management of a baby could not be presumed'.[15]

Although Sefi does not investigate the client's perception of these interactions, a study by McIntosh (1986) investigated the impact of the interactional style of health visitors on a sample of mothers in Scotland.[18] Almost two-thirds of the mothers in this study complained of health visitors being too directive and, as McIntosh (1987) notes: 'the resentment which a directive approach engendered was exceedingly damaging to the health visitor–client relationship and greatly reduced their service's effectiveness'.[19]

Although McIntosh's study relied on the mother's reports of the health visitors' interactional style, it does appear to complement Sefi's findings. Both studies isolated instances of the health visitor adopting an affiliative style or being identified by the client as 'friendly', but these were in the minority. This would also support Rogers and Pilgrim's (unpublished) suggestion that parents whose own expertise is respected and who experience a more affiliative style from their doctor or health visitor are more in favour of the health practitioners.[20] Although Rogers and Pilgrim's sample were a self-selected group, parents from other groups do perceive themselves to have expertise in child-rearing, as indicated by Foster and Mayall's 1990 study in the inner city.[21]

Montgomery-Robinson's (1987) work further elaborated on the nature of the interaction between health visitor and client.[17] She too concentrated on the primary visit and the study is based on 28 such encounters. Unlike Sefi (1985),[15] Montgomery-Robinson places her study firmly in the field of ethnomethodological ethnography, and as such her analytic categories using conversation analysis techniques[16] are derived from the data, and she avoids prejudging her data. She describes her task as not one of judging health visiting but of describing how the participants have defined and displayed health visiting through the selective use and recognition of particular elements of social interaction. In so doing she defined some categories of talk within which the health visitor–client encounter is managed and from which some inferences may be drawn. An example of one of Montgomery-Robinson's defined elements of social interaction is the 'extended turn' – this usually consisted of an explanation or monologue by the health visitor or an account or story by the client, although story-telling was rare. She suggests that differential use of such features means that, although they may contribute equal amounts of talk, the participants are not contributing equally to the interaction. Another element of the interaction was closure and on this point the author notes that 'the lack of an explicit agenda, coupled with an understanding on the part of the mothers that the health visitor has some plan or purpose, makes it very difficult for the mothers to predict when closing is likely to occur'.[17]

These observations would suggest a controlling role by the health visitor and the author does describe an asymmetrical relationship. Montgomery-Robinson also makes observations on the role of other family members, suggesting that the limited contribution of fathers and grandmothers and their expectation that the mother and baby would be the focus of attention implies that in many cases the concept of the *family* visitor cannot be upheld.

Kendall's 1991 study[22] of health visitor–client interactions supports the findings of both Sefi and Montgomery-Robinson. Kendall's study differed from the earlier two as the sample consisted of mothers with children under 1 year of age, but excluded the primary visit on the grounds that this was in many ways atypical. The sample was also larger (75) and included families from two quite different health authorities. An additional component was the interview data collected from both clients and health visitors as referred to previously. Again using conversation analysis, Kendall found evidence of control of the interactions by the health visitor supported by features such as the way advice was given, gathering and providing information, and closure of the interaction. Most notably, of 350 sequences of advice giving, 95% were apparently unsolicited by the mothers. This led to a didactic approach to advice giving with little participation by the mothers or acknowledgment of their expertise as mothers or in any other capacity. As discussed above, these findings were supported by an analysis of interviews with the mothers following the visits. Immunisation was frequently on the health visitor's agenda, but was not clear to the client.

SUMMARY

- The style and nature of the professional–client interaction often constrains the possibility of clients making informed decisions.

- Professionals tend to control the interaction.

- There is a tendency for professionals to give advice rather then elicit concerns from clients.

- Factors such as time, socio-economic group and ethnicity may be important variables in the negotiation process.

- There is little evidence of a theoretical framework for health promotion underpinning the interaction.

References

1. Roter, D., Hall, J., Katz, N. 'Patient–physician communication – a descriptive summary of the literature', *Patient Education and Counselling*, 1988; 12: 99–119.

2. Johnson, W.L., Hardin, C.A. *Content and dynamics of home visits of public health nurses. Part I.* 1962. American Nurses Foundation New York Inc.

3. Clark, J. 'Recording health visitor/client interaction in home visits', *Health Visitor*, 1984; 75: 5–8.

4. Byrne, P., Long, B. *Doctors talking to patients.* 1976. HMSO, London.

5. Baldock, J., Prior, D. 'Social workers talking to clients – a study of verbal behaviour', *British Journal of Social Work*, 1981; 11: 19–38.

6. Tuckett, D., Olson, C., Williams, A., Booth, M. *The Patient Project.* 1982. Health Education Studies Unit, Health Education Council, London.

7. Macleod-Clark, J. 'Nurse–patient verbal interactions: a study of conversations on selected surgical wards'. 1982. Unpublished Ph.D. thesis, University of London.

8. Clifton, J. 'Social workers talking to clients – a comment', *British Journal of Social Work*, 1981; 11: 39–42.

9. Tuckett, D., Bolton, M., Olson, C. and Williams, A. *Meetings between experts.* 1985. Tavistock, London.

10. Health Visitors' Association. *Health visiting and school nursing – the future.* 1985. HVA, London.

11. Warner, U. 'Asking the right questions', *Nursing Times, Community Outlook*, 1984; 13 June: 214–16.

12. Freeman, S. 'Health promotion talk in family practice encounters', *Social Science & Medicine*, 1987; 25(8): 961–6.

13. Arnston, P., Philipsborn, H. 'Paediatrician–parent communication in a continuity of care setting', *Clinical Paediatrics*, 1982; 21(5): 302–7.

14. Street, R. 'Communicative styles and adaptations in physician–parent consultations', *Social Science & Medicine*, 1992; 34(10): 1155–63.

15. Sefi, S. 'The first visit: a study of health visitor/mother verbal interaction'. 1985. Unpublished MA dissertation, University of Warwick.

16. Heritage, J. *Garfinkel and ethnomethodology.* 1984. Polity Press, Cambridge.

17. Montgomery-Robinson, K. 'The social construction of health visiting'. 1987. Unpublished Ph.D. thesis, Polytechnic of the South Bank, London.

18. McIntosh, J. *A consumer perspective on the health visiting service.* 1986. Social and Paediatric Research Unit, University of Glasgow.

19. McIntosh, J. 'Interpersonal style and professional effectiveness', *Focus*, 1987; 7: 6–8.

20. Rogers, A., Pilgrim, D. 'Non-compliance with childhood immunisation: personal accounts of parents and health care professionals' Unpublished.

21. Foster, M.C., Mayall, B. 'Health visitors as educators', *Journal of Advanced Nursing*, 1990; 15: 286–92.

22. Kendall, S. The influence of the health visiting process on client participation: an analysis of the health visitor–client interaction. 1991. Unpublished Ph.D. thesis, King's College London.

8. Sources of information about immunisation

Research investigating information used by health professionals will be reviewed here, together with a consideration of some sources of information that are currently available for use by health professionals as well as parents.

INFORMATION USED BY HEALTH PROFESSIONALS

A national study to investigate the variation in uptake of immunisation between districts and to identify those procedures closely linked with high uptake was undertaken for the DoH in 1989.[1] Interviews were conducted with all the immunisation coordinators (response rate 93%) and postal questionnaires were sent to 1070 health visitors in 21 districts. Despite a relatively low response rate of 64% (689) from the health visitors, the study provides useful information on a number of issues and is one of the few studies to have investigated sources of information for health professionals.

- Overall, 95% of the health visitors responding felt either very well or fairly well informed about immunisation.

- Most of the health visitors assessed the practical and formal training they had received about immunisation as being adequate. Three out of five had received in-service training within the last year. (MMR vaccine was introduced during this period, so it is to be expected that some training would have been provided.)

- 83% had been issued with their own copy of the DoH memorandum on immunisation; 85% of these said they found it very useful, but a small number (6%) claimed never to use it.

- 69% had been issued with a copy of the district's guidelines, but it was much more likely for health visitors in high uptake districts to have these guidelines than those in low uptake districts (84% vs 67%). Also, 10% did not know whether their district had its own guidelines. Of the 352 health visitors who had their own copy of district guidelines, 92% indicated they found it very useful.

- In terms of information given to parents, HEA leaflets were almost universally used, with 98% of respondents claiming to use them. The health visitors found the leaflets more effective if used as a basis for discussion and thought they would be improved if they contained more detail and information.

In a survey of 107 Oxfordshire health visitors in 1987, sources of information which they used for queries about immunisation were investigated.[2] Some source of reference was listed by 96%, with most using a variety – the most commonly used written sources were the clinic policy handbook (28%) and district health authority leaflets – while only 18% claimed to use the DoH memorandum. This is in contrast with findings in 1994 that 88% of 54 health professionals said they had read the DoH memorandum and 60% claimed to have read all of it.[3] This finding is probably partly due to an increased awareness and commitment to immunisation that has developed over the past years and to the publication of a more user-friendly, useful and informative document from the DoH.

SOURCES OF INFORMATION ABOUT IMMUNISATION

This section describes some of the sources of information about immunisation that are currently available. This is by no means an exhaustive review and does not include the many textbooks and chapters dealing with the subject, although some of these are listed at the end of the references in this chapter. In addition, numerous papers and articles are published in the medical and nursing press every week.

Handbooks

Immunisation against infectious disease (DoH, 1996)[4]

This handbook is the definitive guide to immunisation and is probably the most widely available source of information for use by health professionals. It is circulated to all doctors in England, District Immunisation Coordinators, Directors of Public Health, medical and nursing officers, health visitors, pharmacists, general managers at regional and district level, and Family Health Services Authorities (FHSA). It can also be purchased in HMSO and other bookshops.

The handbook provides detailed information on immunisation procedures, the epidemiology of each of the vaccine-preventable diseases, and information about the vaccines and their indications, contraindications and adverse reactions. Now updated at approximately two-year intervals, it provides a practical guide to immunisation. Although it is clear and straightforward to use, the language employed is for a medical readership; however, it is not intended to be used widely by parents.

Immunizing children (Mayon-White and Moreton, 1997)[5]

This practical guide to immunisation was written for those directly involved in providing immunisation and is also intended to be comprehensible to parents. In addition to information on the vaccine-preventable diseases, schedule for immunisation, and immunisation procedure, it contains a section dealing with specific medical circumstances and another containing answers to questions most frequently asked by parents.

Guidelines produced by health authorities

In addition to these publications, individual districts and FHSAs have produced their own guidelines. These are too numerous to be considered individually; it was reported in 1987 that 154 districts had produced their own formal policy[6] and it is likely that this figure has increased more recently. The guidelines generally tend to adopt a similar format; for example Nottingham Health Authority has produced a practical guide that deals with most of the queries arising in practice and counters the more common myths. Locally produced guidelines are particularly useful as they are able to include local information such as policies, vaccine advisory clinics, and information on whom to contact for advice. However, it is important that they are compatible with the memorandum from the DoH.[7]

Special advisory services

A number of districts have established vaccine advisory services, whose aim is not only to investigate and advise on immunisation in relation to specific medical problems but also to influence immunisation uptake in the community through education and demonstration of good practice. Over a two-year period, 191 children attended the advisory service in Clwyd and most referrals related to pertussis vaccine.[8] Immunisation did not proceed in only ten cases and there were no reports of untoward reactions. Similar impressive results have been reported by Ko *et al.* (1995).[9] Some districts have established immunisation telephone 'hotlines' available for use by health professionals who have a query about immunisation. These are often set up on a temporary basis to accompany the introduction of a new vaccine.

Vaccine manufacturers' data sheets

All packs of vaccine contain manufacturer's instructions. Little is known about the extent to which these are used as a source of information although it is thought that, along with other information provided by drug companies, they may be used widely by practice nurses (*personal communication* – Community Health Adviser, Royal College of Nursing [RCN]). In 1984, Hull and Nicoll pointed out that the recommendations from the DHSS, the British National Formulary and manufacturers' inserts were not in accord with one another and urged manufacturers to bring their guidance in line with official policy.[10] This has also been commented on by Stevens and Baker (1989)[11] and Elliman (1990)[12] who highlighted the inconsistencies in advice from the *Data sheet compendium* and *Monthly index of medical specialties (MIMS)*, pointing out that many doctors use these publications. The situation has still not been rectified and the contraindications listed for Trivax triple antigen in the 1994 edition of *MIMS* remain at variance with DoH recommendations.

Training materials

A number of training packs relate to immunisation and are an extremely effective means of increasing and updating health professionals' knowledge about immunisation. Their primary intention is not as a means of teaching communication skills and so they do not fulfil this purpose.

Mukerjee (1994) reported findings from an audit of Hib immunisation training sessions in Mid Glamorgan.[13] Training sessions were held using the materials produced by the Welsh Office (similar to the DoH materials). An immunisation enquiry telephone hotline was also established and during the three months after the launch of the vaccine all enquiries about Hib vaccine received from primary health care professionals were documented. A review of the nature of these enquiries indicated that non-attendance for training sessions was associated with a lack of knowledge, particularly about dose schedules. Mukerjee concludes that training sessions could be a crucial factor in determining district uptake rates and that written guidelines alone cannot replace the sessions.

The Nottingham training pack

In response to concern about areas of extremely low immunisation uptake, Nottingham Health Authority developed a training procedure for health professionals. This comprises a training manual with explicit instructions for the trainer and a video plus a practical guide for the individual practitioner. The half-day training session is conducted in an informal atmosphere and includes practical and theoretical aspects of immunisation, together with a session of role play where a health professional counsels a parent who has specific concerns about immunisation. The authors comment that pertussis immunisation causes health professionals the most anxiety.

A group of 47 health visitors attending a refresher course undertook the training procedure and, when assessed pre- and post-training, were found to have improved knowledge and certainty about immunisation. This improvement was maintained when they were assessed six months later. In addition, immunisation rates improved in Nottingham Health Authority during the period of the training initiative. Nottingham has organised training days for trainers from other health authorities and the procedure has been used widely by many districts.

Vaccines in general practice **(Royal College of Nursing, 1993)**[14]

The Community Nursing Advisory section of the RCN is frequently contacted by community nurses, particularly practice nurses, who have queries about immunisation. In response to this expressed need for more information, and recognising that practice nurses have a major role in the provision of immunisation in general practice, the RCN has held 60 seminars across the country. The programme is designed to offer nurses a forum for the exchange of ideas and discussion of current issues, together with an opportunity to learn more about the provision of immunisation. The content of the information pack that accompanies the programme has been informed by discussion with 200 practice nurses about their concerns. It is intended to publish a stand-alone handbook based on the material in the information pack. The main focus of the programme is on adult/travel immunisation although childhood immunisation is considered. No evaluation of this new initiative is available yet.

Hib vaccine information pack (DoH/HEA, 1992)[15]

Prior to the introduction of Hib vaccine the DoH and HEA produced information for health professionals and parents about the new vaccine. This included a leaflet providing guidance for health professionals on answering parents' questions, a question and answer leaflet for health professionals, detailed information on the disease and vaccine extracted from the DoH memorandum on immunisation (1992),[16] and a leaflet for parents.

HEA campaigns

Immunisation campaign, 1994

In 1994 the HEA campaign focused on immunisation in general and included the production of an updated pamphlet for parents entitled *A guide to childhood immunisations*, together with advertisements on television and in the press and posters. The leaflet contains more information than earlier versions, particularly about the side-effects of immunisation, and also includes a section on recognising meningitis. It is available in 20 languages.

The campaign included one advertisement which depicts a scan-type image of a child's head with damaged areas of the brain; the caption reads: 'And you thought measles only caused little marks on the skin'. Like other adverts used in the campaign, reactions to this were pre-tested among 20 parents either in in-depth interviews or group discussions.[17] While it is true that measles can cause brain damage, it is a rare complication. It has been suggested that health education messages that are designed to provoke fear and encourage uptake of a health action such as immunisation or cessation of smoking need to relate to adverse events, such as complications of diseases, which are likely to occur in the absence of immunisation.[18]

School-based measles/rubella campaign, 1994

Following a rapid increase in the incidence of measles among school-aged children, the Joint Committee on Vaccination and Immunisation (JCVI) recommended that a school-based campaign to prevent a predicted epidemic of measles should be scheduled for November 1994. The materials produced by the HEA to support this campaign comprised a leaflet containing a consent form for parents, translated into ten languages, together with television advertising. The television advert delivered a powerful message: measles is serious and can kill or cause serious complications such as brain damage. Fact sheets were also produced for the press and public relations. Feature articles were written for newspapers and magazines with almost all family and mother and baby magazines running articles on measles and/or immunisation during the period of the campaign.

Information generally available for health professionals included papers in the medical and nursing press, a circular from the DoH in a question and answer format, and a special unit of the RCN's continuing education project, which included a television programme screened on BBC Select.

The measles/rubella campaign was a success, with 92% vaccine coverage and few subsequent cases of laboratory-confirmed measles infection.[19] Evaluation of the campaign was conducted in two waves by the HEA. In the post-immunisation programme wave more than 3 in 5 of 748 mothers of 5–15-year-olds who were interviewed claimed to have heard or seen advertising, information or publicity about immunisation in the previous 12 months. The most likely source of information was television advertising. Attitudes to this were quite positive, although 58% of those who had consulted their own doctor for information found it very helpful compared with 31% of those who obtained information from television advertising.[20]

Despite the success of the campaign there were some criticisms, notably that the information about vaccine side-effects contained in the leaflet for parents was inadequate[21] and that the television advertising traded on individuals' fears and portrayed measles as a much more serious disease than is the reality.

Alternative literature/literature from lay organisations

This section is not intended to provide an exhaustive review of sources of alternative literature. Some have already been considered in the section on homeopathy.

What Doctors Don't Tell You (WDDTY, 1991)[22]

This publication is edited by a journalist, reports on 'dangerous or questionable drugs, surgery or investigative tests' and is generally anti-medicine on all fronts. A vaccination handbook has been produced with the subtitle *A guide to the dangers of childhood immunisation* which pulls together all the 'evidence' that WDDTY has amassed about immunisation. Using the same techniques as Chaitow and Coulter and taking selective quotes from scientific sources, they claim 'together these writings make an unabashed case against vaccination'. It appears to be effective in convincing some parents not to proceed with immunisation, as one mother commented: 'the copy you sent me persuaded me not to have my daughter vaccinated any more after she reacted to her first jabs'.[22]

An example of the type of approach taken by WDDTY followed a report in *The New England Journal of Medicine* of an acellular pertussis vaccine trial – a randomised, double-blind, placebo-controlled trial conducted in Sweden.[23] Infants were vaccinated with either diphtheria and tetanus vaccine alone (DT, 1726 infants) or with diphtheria, tetanus and pertussis (DTP, 1724 infants) at 3, 5 and 12 months. There were 312 cases of pertussis – 72 in the DTP group and 240 in the DT group – a vaccine efficacy of 55% after two doses and 71% after three doses. No serious reactions to the vaccines were reported. Two infants in the DTP group had febrile convulsions within 48 hours of the third vaccination; both had respiratory tract infections. One child with pneumococcal endocarditis in the DTP group died. Four children in the DT group had invasive bacterial infections, and all recovered. Five children developed malignant disease, two in the DTP group and three in the DT group.

The *WDDTY* report of this paper was entitled 'Pertussis jab: half effective'.[24] This report mentioned the reactions but excluded the details that the children who suffered convulsions also had respiratory tract infections, that the child who died had endocarditis, that the children with bacterial infections recovered, or that the children with cancer were in both vaccine groups. Further, the number of cases of pertussis is quoted as 321 (not 312) and it is not made clear that 77% of these cases occurred in the group who did not receive the pertussis vaccine. The authors state: 'Researchers claim the vaccine to be 71% efficacious, although this fell to 55% after the second shot. In other words, it is only half effective.'[24]

It is not clear if it was the intention of the authors of this piece to misrepresent the original paper or whether they have misunderstood the findings. Clearly, this kind of reporting does not assist parents who need accurate information about immunisation and may not have access to the original source.

The Informed Parent

The Informed Parent is the newsletter of the parents' organisation of the same name which was established in 1992. The organisation has over 1000 members and aims to promote awareness and understanding about immunisation and its alternatives and to enable parents to make an informed choice, supporting them whatever their choice. The newsletter aims to provide parents with information which is both pro- and anti-immunisation. For example, in issue 5 (October 1993) a letter was published from the neighbour of a child who died aged 6 months as a result of Hib meningitis. She describes the fear that struck communities in her youth following a case of diphtheria and polio and the damage caused by whooping cough and measles. Printed on the opposite page was a review of Hib vaccine. The severity of meningitis is described but it also states that Hib infections are not common in childhood and children living in deprived communities are at greater risk. Using a quotation, it is also suggested that excessive use of drugs and vaccinations impairs the infant's immune system and that, because of the impaired state of health that results from receiving the traditional set of vaccinations, another vaccine, that is, Hib, had to be introduced.

More recently, the content of the newsletter has tended to focus on the risks of immunisation. In January 1996 a paper discussing rubella vaccination was reprinted from another journal first published in 1982. The article began with the sentence: 'The rubella vaccination programme has failed. This is the conclusion of a recent study carried out in Glasgow.' The paper was referring to a vaccination programme which has been discontinued and to a vaccine which is no longer used, but these considerations were not made clear in the *Informed Parent* article.[25]

The power of the anecdote

The Informed Parent uses anecdotal cases to support its arguments. One headline was: '**Devastated family** – Little Michaela Neighbour was a golden-haired, adorable little girl ... until, that is, she was given her MMR shot.'

This kind of approach can be extremely powerful, and trades on an individual's fear of the possible effects of immunisation on their own loved child; parents may be able to empathise with stories about individual children rather than with the overall picture of the programme.

Newspapers and women's magazines

The media is consistently identified as being an important source of information for parents about immunisation.[26–8] Unfortunately its influence is often negative. In a study of parents who had not consented to immunisation, 30% stated it was because of negative influences from the television and radio and 25% from magazines.[29] At the time of the pertussis controversy in the 1970s there was compelling evidence of the impact of the media on the uptake of the vaccine.

Harding's 1985 study of 253 articles from eight British national daily and eight Sunday newspapers showed that the articles gave a limited amount of information about the diseases and tended to describe the negative aspects of the immunisations.[30] The emphasis was on events concerning individuals rather than programmes or policies. She argues that the press must present a story that is newsworthy and this is best achieved by concentrating on events which are negative, abnormal, involve trouble or conflict, and can be personified. Concentrating on rare events creates a disproportionate perception of risk. These criticisms could also be levelled at much of the literature produced by the anti-immunisation movement.

The wider impact of the media is also important as it may influence attitudes not only among parents who are deciding whether to have a child immunised but also among their friends and relatives who in turn may be asked for advice or opinion. Health professionals, too, may be influenced by these sources.[31]

The ten top-selling women's magazines were reviewed for their coverage of immunisation at the time of the introduction of Hib vaccine in 1992. Most magazines provided brief information about the new vaccine, the effects of the disease and advice to contact the GP or health visitor for further information. More recently *Bella* magazine (the second best-seller) published a feature-length article which included accounts of an 18-year-old boy thought to be brain damaged by pertussis vaccine and a 63-year-old woman who had chronic chest problems due to whooping cough in childhood and who had a daughter born with congenital rubella syndrome. *Bella* also published a piece in their 'Doctor's surgery' section in which a practising GP described a 'real-life' situation where he advised parents of an 8-week-old baby about immunisation.

The magazines reviewed tend to adopt a responsible attitude to immunisation, presenting balanced advice. This supports the findings of Harding (1985), who compared the coverage of immunisation by Britain's quality and popular press and found that, in general, the popular press tended to display a more responsible attitude towards immunisation.[32] For example, she found they were more likely to name parents as being responsible for immunisation and to suggest seeking the advice of health professionals.

Articles with an anti-immunisation flavour have been published in the quality press.[33–5] Tyler takes a particularly strong one-sided anti-immunisation line, describing the HEA's publications as 'scandalously complacent' and the DoH memorandum as including data which are 'elaborately skewed to make the immunisation programme look safer and more effective than it really is'.[33] Tyler cites the work of Coulter, and Richard Moskowitz, an American homeopathic GP, and provides no information in support of immunisation.

Television

A number of television programmes are considered here.

Channel 4, *Dispatches*, 'The batches in question' (17 November 1993)

This programme told the story of a mother's determination in winning the right of access to documents held by the Wellcome Foundation and then wading through them looking for crucial evidence that might explain her son's severe brain damage following pertussis vaccine. She found a document which conceded that the re-analysis of tests on the relevant batch of vaccine suggested it to be toxic and that the company would not have permitted its release today. This resulted in the award of £2.75 million damages from Wellcome to the 24-year-old man with severe impairments.

The programme also investigated the circumstances in several other cases associated with batches produced at the same time as the toxic batch. The programme implied that, even if pertussis vaccine were the cause of brain damage, in these cases it related to vaccines produced more than 20 years ago.

This was a moving and triumphant story for the mother whose son was awarded damages. Unfortunately, any programme of this nature could have an adverse effect on the immunisation programme and cause anxiety for parents.

3D (14 April 1994)

This programme focused on the parents' group JABS which has been set up by parents who consider their children to have been damaged by MMR. The founder member made it clear that the group are not opposed to immunisation but, because they consider there to be a small but real risk of serious side-effects attached to MMR vaccine, parents should be provided with all the available information, including the chance of serious side-effects. A lawyer featured on the programme pointed out that, owing to the financial incentive for GPs to reach immunisation targets, some parents feel they are under pressure to have their children immunised, and in these circumstances it is particularly important that they are aware of all the benefits and risks of immunisation.

Several families whose children were said to have developed serious problems after receiving MMR vaccine were featured. It was implied that parents had been given little or no information about the side-effects of immunisation and, in cases where information had been provided, it was suggested that side effects were only ever minor. As there was no opportunity for any discussion about the likely cause of these children's problems or about the risk attached to natural infection, it is likely that this programme will have caused many parents considerable anxiety.

World in Action, 'A shot in the dark' (28 November 1994)

In addition to the considerable news coverage, a number of programmes were screened during and shortly after the 1994 school-based measles/rubella immunisation campaign. The issues raised in the *World in Action* programme were concerned with the rationale for the measles/rubella campaign, the suggestion that the vaccine is not as effective as is thought, that adverse events following vaccination are unacknowledged and under-reported, and that some children were being immunised without their parents' consent. Members of JABS, a lawyer for JABS and immunisation experts were featured.

The flavour of the programme was critical of the campaign and, although the case for immunisation was covered, the medical establishment in general was seen as aloof and unlistening.

BBC2, *Esther* (30 January 1996)

This programme has a studio-discussion format. The audience comprised three health professionals who support the vaccination programme and two who have been openly critical, members of parents' organisations who consider their children to have been vaccine-damaged, individuals who had been damaged by the diseases, and representatives from WDDTY, The Informed Parent and JABS. The main thrust was the lack of information for parents about possible side-effects surrounding the measles/rubella campaign. Since the majority of the audience were critical of the immunisation programme the balance was in that direction.

It is unlikely that, viewed individually, any of these programmes would have a very damaging effect on the immunisation programme by encouraging parents to reject immunisation. However, they bring some of the more extreme views against immunisation to the attention of a wide audience and, taken together and along with some of the articles in the quality press, could result in raising the anxiety of many parents. It is important that the health professionals who advise parents about immunisation are aware of the content of these programmes and newspaper articles and are prepared to discuss the issues raised.

COMMUNICATION TRAINING MATERIALS

Counselling or counselling skills have been referred to as the qualities and abilities necessary for any health care professional to help people, whatever their problem and whatever the specialty.[36] These skills are needed to communicate in the consultation situation where there are three basic requirements:

- at least two people should be involved;
- the aim is for one of these people to help the other (one seeking advice, the other attempting to provide it);
- there must be at least minimal or tacit agreement about the nature of their interaction.

The evidence reviewed suggests that the latter two of these basic requirements for enabling communication are often not fulfilled in relation to consultation about immunisation. The resulting lack of communication leads to dissatisfaction, poor understanding of the issues surrounding immunisation, and in some cases rejection of immunisation and primary health care in general.

A variety of training methods have been employed in an attempt to improve the communication skills of health workers. Apart from the Nottingham training procedure and the HEA (1990) programme[37] designed along the same lines as the Nottingham pack, there are no training materials designed for primary health care workers which specifically deal with communication and counselling in relation to immunisation. Numerous training materials focus on communication and counselling skills for particular groups, for example nurses,[38] or for specific subjects such as depression.[39] An analysis of all the materials is not possible in this review, but key points that have emerged from evaluation of training procedures will be considered.

Evaluation of communication skills courses for health professionals demonstrates that they are successful in improving the ability to communicate with patients and clients.[40,41] Fielding and Llewelyn (1987) consider that a number of components are essential for effective communication training.[42]

- A need for improved communication must be identified. This review has demonstrated this need in relation to immunisation.

- Good communication must be desired by health organisations. For example, with respect to immunisation, encouraging clients to ask questions may be threatening for health professionals as it may reveal gaps in their knowledge. It is clear that some parents require detailed information and ask searching questions. Training which incorporates role play is a useful approach as it not only provides guidance on counselling but can also increase confidence and knowledge about immunisation. The use of video in role play has been found to be particularly effective as a method of feedback.

- The organisation must support a particular individual when trained. There is evidence that any changes brought about in individuals during training are quickly nullified and reversed by their re-entry to the organisation.[42]

In order to minimise this possibility in relation to training focusing on consultation about immunisation, the setting for training and the participants are briefly considered below.

It is clear that the provision of immunisation is dependent on individuals from a variety of disciplines including nursing, medical and clerical staff. Recommendations for conducting the Nottingham training procedure suggested that nursing and medical staff should be trained separately; it was found that, if the two professional groups were mixed, nurses did not derive the same educational value from their attendance because they tended to defer to the doctors' opinion.[43] However, as teamwork is regarded as essential for effective health promotion in the primary care setting[44] and as consistency of information offered is also crucial, training within the primary health care team may be desirable. Fundamental problems are associated with multidisciplinary training in some districts. In Liverpool health visitors are employed by one trust, CMOs and the immunisation coordinator by another trust, and two-thirds of immunisations are given in general practice.[45]

A paper discussing issues relating to developments in general practice considered that the developments which include arrangements for practices to contract for community nursing and health visiting services will enable multidisciplinary learning to come into its own, with in-house training for doctors and nurses linked to practice-based quality-improving exercises.[46] Joint training programmes for health authority nurses and practice nurses to encourage joint working and understanding among the nursing groups have also been recommended.[44] The inclusion of doctors may have wider benefits by increasing appreciation of each other's roles and breaking down barriers to communication between disciplines.

A major obstacle to training in communication skills emerged from a study of 620 practice nurses in South West Thames Regional Health Authority.[47] It was found that, although the majority of nurses surveyed wanted to develop their role in communication skills/counselling and health promotion, when a course was provided and advertised so few nurses applied that the course was cancelled. Telephone interviews were conducted with 18 nurses who had expressed an interest in the course but who had not applied to ascertain the reasons for poor take-up. Of these, ten said that their employing GP had not considered it to be a priority, with comments such as 'you should know about communicating by now' and the course was 'too wishy-washy'. This adds further support to the provision of training within the practice team setting.

Any training in communication skills designed by the HEA would be best promoted with the focus on immunisation rather than on communication skills as this may be perceived as too vague. It may be difficult for individuals to recognise they have a need for communication skills training. Achieving and maintaining targets for immunisation, however, are incentives for many practices and an opportunity to consider and critically review their approach to immunisation is likely to be a priority.

Finally, it is important that training is set within a theoretical framework using issues about immunisation as a method of highlighting theories, processes and communication skills. The skills thus acquired can then be generalised and applied to other situations. It has been observed that, without a framework, training tends to drift from method to method, allowing the techniques to become ends in themselves, with little understanding of the meaning and purpose of what is being attempted.[41]

Two different approaches adopted in training packages will be considered, one utilising a passive approach where communication techniques are taught by watching actors role-playing on video, and a second where the techniques are taught and participants engage in role-play themselves. Video recordings are used as a method of feedback.

Defeating depression

A video teaching package, *Depression: from recognition to management*,[39] has been produced to support the first phase of the national campaign to defeat depression, focusing on professional knowledge and skills. The teaching pack emphasises practical demonstrations of the skills and so video is used as an effective training resource. Some aspects of the approach and format used could be a useful model for the development of training materials for communication skills relating to immunisation.

The pack has been designed for small group teaching. Videotaped sessions aim at drawing attention to the skills required to identify depressive illness. The video uses a traditional format of studio discussion with acted-out scenarios depicting good and bad practice. Case-studies are used to illustrate a shift from 'doctor-centred' to 'patient-centred' approaches and the key communication skills which facilitate this are identified, including how to pick up on cues and encourage patients to discuss feelings.

Microtraining

Crute *et al.* (1989) describe an evaluation of a communication skills training course for health visitor students, designed to develop the health visitor's ability to communicate with clients.[40] The programme utilised the microtraining method, one of the best researched and most systematic approaches,[48] which involves four phases.

- The analysis of skills in terms of their functions, behavioural components and discussion of related findings.

- Training participants to critically evaluate skill use in terms of discriminating effective and ineffective employment of skills.

- Practice in adopting these skills in video-recorded role-play situations of health visitor–client interactions.

- Feedback through replay of recordings and tutor and peer evaluation.

The training programme focused upon several skill areas which had been identified by the organisers as relevant to health visitor goals in social interaction, including non-verbal behaviour, reinforcement, questioning, reflecting, explaining, and opening and closing interaction.

The sample group for the evaluation was composed of 31 health visitor students. The microtraining programme lasted eight weeks and comprised a two-hour lecture and a three-hour practical session each week. Effectiveness of the programme in improving trainees' interpersonal skills was examined by assessing trainee social behaviour in a relevant professional situation both before and following training.

The training programme had limitations which are described in detail by the authors. In spite of these the training programme was successful in improving the students' social competence. For example, during the post-training role play, health visitor students used significantly more communicative gestures and encouraged client response more than before training. They also received higher scores for explaining, and opening and closure skills.

The authors comment that this training approach requires more validation among health visitors but that it has been employed in the education of many professional groups including counsellors, medical students, nurses, nurse teachers, social workers, physiotherapists and speech and language therapists.

References

1. British Market Research Bureau. 'The uptake of pre-school immunisation in England'. 1989. Unpublished report for the Department of Health.

2. Robertson, C.M., Bennett, V.J. 'Health visitor's views on immunisation', *Health Visitor*, 1987; 60: 221–2.

3. Alderson, P., Mayall, B., Barker, S., Henderson, J., Pratten, B. 'Childhood immunisation: support to health professionals' in Hey, V. (ed.) *Immunisation research: a summary volume.* 1997. HEA, London.

4. Department of Health. *Immunisation against infectious disease.* 1996. HMSO, London.

5. Mayon-White, R. and Moreton, J. *Immunizing children – a practical guide.* 1997. Radcliffe Medical Press, Oxford.

6. Begg, N., White, J. 'A survey of pre-school immunisation programmes in England and Wales', *Community Medicine* 1988 10: 344–56.

7. Nicoll, A., Elliman, D., Begg, N.T. 'Immunisation: causes of failure and strategies and tactics for success', *British Medical Journal*, 1989; 299: 808–12.

8. Hall, R., Williams, A.L.J. 'Special advisory service for immunisation', *Archives of Disease in Childhood*, 1988; 63: 1498–1500.

9. Ko, M.L.B., Rao, M., Taere, L., Bridgman, G.C.B., Kurian, A. 'Outcome of referrals to a district immunisation advisory clinic', *Communicable Disease Report*, 1995; 5(10): R146–R149.

10. Hull, D., Nicoll, A. 'Immunisation misinformation' (letter), *The Lancet*, 1984; ii: 1215–16.

11. Stevens, D., Baker, R. 'Parents' beliefs about vaccination', *British Medical Journal*, 1989; 299: 257.

12. Elliman, D. 'Vaccinations and professional confusion' (letter), *British Medical Journal*, 1990; 301: 551.

13. Mukerjee, A. 'An audit of *Haemophilus influenzae* b (Hib) immunisation training sessions in Mid Glamorgan' (letter), *Journal of Public Health Medicine*, 1994; 16(1): 118–19.

14. Royal College of Nursing. *Vaccines in general practice.* 1993. Royal College of Nursing, London.

15. Department of Health/Health Education Authority. 'Hib vaccine information pack'. 1992. Department of Health, London.

16. Department of Health. *Immunisation against infectious disease.* 1992. HMSO, London.

17. Health Education Authority. 'Childhood immunisation advertising campaign'. 1993. Unpublished report for the HEA, London.

18. Soames-Job, R.F. 'Effective and ineffective use of fear in health promotion campaigns', *American Journal of Public Health*, 1988; 78(2): 163–7.

19. Department of Health. 'Measles, rubella (MR) immunisation campaign 1994: one year on.' *CMO's Update*, 1995; 8:1.

20. Health Education Authority. 'Measles-rubella immunisation campaign'. 1995. Project report and evaluation. Unpublished.

21. Unauthored. 'Spotlight on measles', *The Informed Parent*, 1995; 10: 1.

22. What Doctors Don't Tell You. *The WDDTY vaccination handbook.* 1991. Wallace Press, London.

23. Trollfors, B., Taranger, J., Lagerard, T., Lind, L., Sundh, V., Zackerisson, G. *et al.* 'A placebo-controlled trial of a pertussis-toxoid vaccine', *The New England Journal of Medicine*, 1995; 333(16): 1045–50.

24. What Doctors Don't Tell You. 'Pertussis jab: half effective', *What Doctors Don't Tell You*, 1995; December. p. 4.

25. Nightingale, M. 'Rubella vaccination: a failure', *The Informed Parent*, 1996: January.

26. Peckham, C., Bedford, H., Senturia, Y., Ades, A. *National Immunisation Study: factors influencing immunisation uptake in childhood.* 1989. Action Research, Horsham.

27. Gill, E., Sutton, S. 'Immunisation uptake: the role of parental attitudes' in Hey, V. (ed.) *Immunisation research: a summary volume.* 1998. HEA, London.

28. Unpublished HEA data.

29. Reid, J.A. 'Vaccination viewpoints', *Health Visitor*, 1989; 62: 121–3.

30. Harding, C.M. 'Immunisation as depicted by the British National Press' *Community Medicine*, 1985; 7: 87-98.

31. Mayall, B., Foster, M.C. *Child health care: living with children, working for children.* 1989. Heinemann Nursing, Oxford.

32. Harding, C.M. 'A comparison of the coverage of immunisation by Britain's quality and popular press', *Health Education Journal*, 1985; 2: 89–93.

33. Tyler, A. 'Vaccination: the hidden facts', *Evening Standard Magazine*, 1991; September: 74–5.

34. Williams, L. 'A shot in the dark', *Guardian*, 1993; 20 July.

35. Roberts, Y. 'A shot in the dark', *Sunday Times*, 1995; December.

36. Davis, H., Fallowfield, L. *Counselling and communication in health care.* 1991. Wiley, Chichester.

37. Health Education Authority and Department of Health. *A training guide for the providers of immunisation services.* 1990. HEA, London.

38. Scottish Health Education Group. *A guide to running courses for nurses, midwives, health visitors.* 1989.

39. Royal College of Psychiatrists. *Depression: from recognition to management – video training package.* 1993. RCP, London.

40. Crute, V.C., Hargie, O.D.W., Ellis, R.A.F. 'An evaluation of a communication skills course for health visitor students', *Journal of Advanced Nursing*, 1989; 14: 546–52.

41. Frederikson, L., Bull, P. 'An appraisal of the current status of communication skills training in British medical schools', *Social Science & Medicine*, 1992; 34(5): 515–22.

42. Fielding, R.G., Llewelyn, S.P. 'Communication training in nursing may damage your health and enthusiasm: some warnings', *Journal of Advanced Nursing*, 1987; 12: 281–90.

43. Hutchinson, T., Nicoll, A., Polnay, L., Roden, D. 'A training procedure for immunisation', *Health Trends*, 1987; 19: 19–24.

44. Cant, S., Killoran, A. 'Team tactics: a study of nurse collaboration in general practice', *Health Education Journal*, 1993; 52(4): 203–8.

45. Pearson, M. *et al.* 'Reply to letter', *Archives of Disease in Childhood*, 1994; 70: 356.

46. Irvine, D. 'General practice in the 1990s: a personal view on future developments', *British Journal of General Practice*, 1993; 43: 121–5.

47. Ross, F. 'Barriers to learning', *Nursing Times*, 1992; 88(38): 44–5.

48. Hargie, O.D.W., Saunders, C. 'Training professional skills', in Dowrick, P.W., Biggs, S.J. (eds.) *Using video.* 1983. Wiley, London.

Other sources of information about immunisation

Davies, E.G., Elliman, D.A.C., Hart, C.A., Nicoll, A., Rudd, P.T. (eds, for the BPA) *Manual of childhood infections.* 1996. W. B. Saunders, London.

Dudgeon, J.A., Cutting, W.A.M. (eds.) *Immunisation; principles and practice.* 1991. Chapman & Hall Medical, London.

Ingram, M. *Managing immunisation in general practice.* 1995. Radcliffe Medical Press, Oxford.

Plotkin, S.A., Mortimer, E.A. *Vaccines.* 1994. W. B. Saunders, Philadelphia.

9. Conclusions and recommendations

1. The evidence suggests it is important for the immunisation process to be a satisfactory experience for parents that results in them feeling they have made an informed decision which is supported by health professionals. The immunisation process is the first major encounter that many parents have with the primary health care and child health services, and their attitudes to those services will be shaped by this experience. It is evident that a poor experience can not only have a detrimental effect on acceptance of immunisation but also on take-up of other services.

2. The majority of parents consider immunisation to be important and are satisfied with the immunisation service. A minority, however, have serious criticisms which must be addressed. Parents' dissatisfaction relates to inadequate communication and interpersonal skills on the part of health professionals.

3. It is evident that parents want more detailed information about immunisation. The HEA proposes the production of vaccine information leaflets in a question and answer format. The content of any proposed material should be carefully considered, particularly in view of research findings emerging from the USA about vaccine information leaflets currently in use. More research is needed to investigate precisely what information different parents require.

4. Parents need assistance and encouragement to ask health professionals questions. This could be achieved in two ways. First, communication skills training could be provided for health professionals to equip them with the skills necessary to elicit parents' concerns and questions. Secondly, written material for parents could be provided to outline possible questions they could consider and use as a basis for discussion with health professionals. Questions could be incorporated in the vaccine information leaflets and also in the parent-held child health record now used widely in many districts.

5. Consideration should be given to drawing up detailed guidelines on the minimum amount of information about immunisation that all parents should receive before consenting to their child entering the programme.

6. Research is required into the optimum time and methods of giving parents information about immunisation, particularly for first-time parents, as their decisions about immunisation acceptance appear to apply for subsequent children.

7. As immunisation rates continue to improve, those individuals who elect not to have their children immunised will assume greater importance as a group who may need targeting, particularly with information that meets their needs. Research at a national level is needed to quantify the amount of positive rejection among parents and to explore their reasons for this decision on a larger scale. It is important to ensure that they are not basing their decision on misinformation.

8. There is a need for information which specifically addresses the issues raised in the anti-immunisation literature, sets it in context, and discusses the evidence in an impartial way. This could be used by health professionals and distributed to parents when appropriate.

9. At times of adverse publicity about immunisation, it is important that health professionals are provided with all the relevant information as quickly as possible so they are equipped to deal with the questions that will inevitably follow.

10. It is evident that parents are still receiving inconsistent messages from health professionals. Research is required to investigate the level of health professionals' knowledge about immunisation, particularly in view of the developments and changes in the immunisation programme. This information would provide a useful basis for deciding on the content of any proposed communication training skills materials.

11. Any proposed communication skills training materials focusing on immunisation produced by the HEA should be promoted with the emphasis on immunisation rather than communication. Communication training may be perceived by some health professionals as involving vague and obvious issues and as not being a priority.

12. Further research is needed into the sources of information health professionals use, and consideration should be given to formulating mechanisms to ensure that, as far as possible, they provide consistent information.